# Health Care Benefits Overview

## 2015 Edition, Vol. 1

Building on over
50 years of providing
quality health care services
to our nation's Veterans

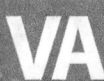 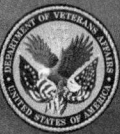

**U.S. Department of Veterans Affairs**
Veterans Health Administration

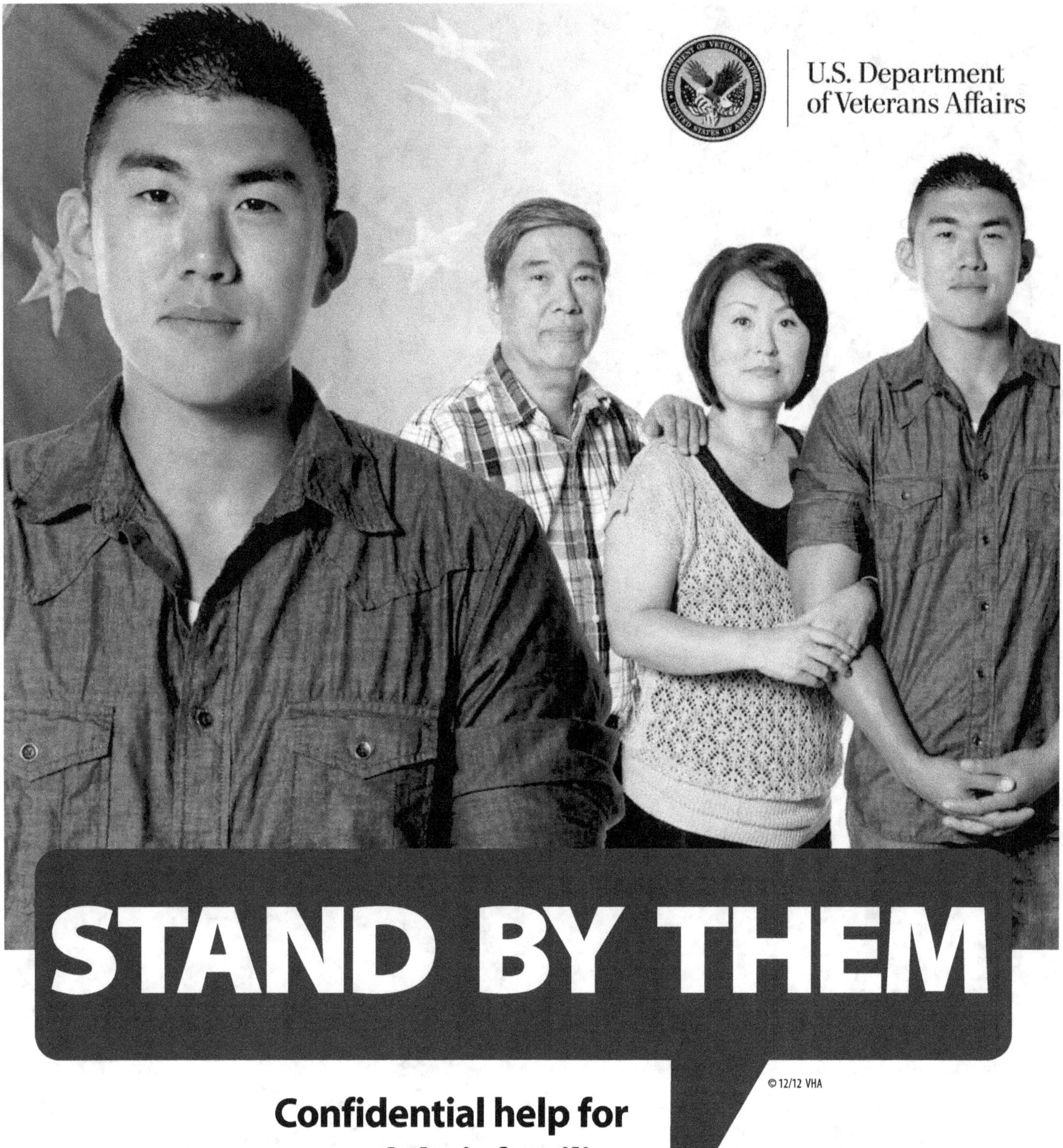

U.S. Department
of Veterans Affairs

# STAND BY THEM

© 12/12 VHA

**Confidential help for
Veterans and their families**

**Veterans
Crisis Line**

# 1-800-273-8255 PRESS ❶

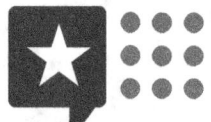

• • • Confidential chat at **VeteransCrisisLine.net** or text to **838255** • • •

# Introduction

This guide is designed to provide Veterans and their families with the information they need to understand VA's health care system—eligibility requirements, the health benefits and services available to help Veterans and copayments that certain Veterans may be charged.

### New Topics and Benefits!

Veterans' Choice Program –See "Non-VA Provider Health Care" on Page 4

The Veteran Health Identification Card (VHIC) - Page 8

Elimination of Annual Means Test (Financial Assessment) – Page 9

Camp Lejeune Eligibility Changes – Page 32

Transportation to VA Appointments – Page 32

Extended Combat Veteran Eligibility - See "What is the Clay Hunt Act" on Page 39

Reporting Health Care Coverage on your Tax Return – Page 42

This book is not intended to provide information on all of the health benefits and services offered by VA. Additional information is available at the following resources:

- www.va.gov/healthbenefits
- VA toll-free 1-877-222-VETS (8387) between 8AM and 8PM ET, Monday - Friday
- Your local VA health care facility's Enrollment Office

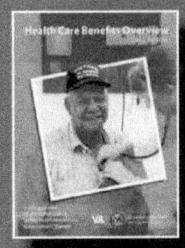

**On the cover:** A doctor listens to Raymond Haskins heart during an appointment at the VA Medical Center located in Washington DC. Mr. Haskins was stationed in Vietnam while serving in the U.S. Army from 1965 to 1967.

# Benefits of Enrolling

Today's Veterans have a comprehensive medical benefits package (see page 21 for a complete list of medical benefits VA offers). The VA offers a variety of health care services from basic primary care to nursing home care for eligible Veterans (see Long-Term Care Standard Benefits section on page 22). If you are enrolled in VA health care, you don't need to take additional steps to meet the healthcare law coverage standards. Enrollment in the VA health care system provides Veterans with the promise that comprehensive health care services will be available when and where they are needed.

In addition to the assurance that services will be available, enrolled Veterans welcome not having to repeat the application process — regardless of where they seek their care or how often. VA is America's largest integrated health care system, serving 8 million Veterans each year.

**Need more reasons to enroll?**

- Medical care rated among the best in the U.S.
- Immediate benefits of health care coverage. Veterans may apply for VA health care enrollment at any time.
- No enrollment fee, monthly premiums, or deductibles. Most Veterans have no out-of- pocket costs. Some Veterans may have to pay small copayments for health care or prescription drugs.
- More than 1,700 places available to get your care. This means your coverage can go with you if you travel or move.
- Freedom to use other plans with your VA health care, including Medicare, Medicaid, TRICARE or private insurance.
- Enrolled Veterans who are traveling or who spend time away from their preferred facility may obtain care at any VA health care facility across the country without the worry of having to reapply.
- Under VA's medical benefits package, the same medical benefits are generally available to all enrolled Veterans.

## Medical Care for Service-Connected Veterans Abroad

Veterans with a VA-rated service-connected condition may receive treatment for that condition even in a foreign country (see Foreign Medical Program on page 33).

## High Quality Care

VA is committed to providing the high quality, safe and effective health care Veterans have earned and deserve. We have established a record of safe, exceptional care that is consistently recognized by independent reviews, organizations and experts. As a result, VA health care performance compares favorably with the Nation on most measures of quality and safety, and patients at VA facilities have comparable or higher satisfaction with VA services to those in non-VA facilities.

For more information visit www.va.gov/qualityofcare/.

## Stay Connected With VA

Share your email address with VA to receive information on VA benefits and services delivered right to your inbox! Visit the "Stay Connected with VA" box located on VA's homepage at www.va.gov and enter your email address to start receiving information about VA benefits.

# VA Health Care Enrollment and Eligibility

## Quickly Find Out If You May Be Eligible For Enrollment

Use the online VA Health Benefits Explorer at hbexplorer.vacloud.us to answer a few questions about yourself (you will be asked no more than 15 questions) and learn about the VA health care benefits you could receive as an enrolled Veteran. Afterwards, you will be given an opportunity to apply for enrollment. If you wish, you may skip the Explorer and simply apply for enrollment using one of the options below.

### Ways to Apply for Enrollment

There are four ways to apply for enrollment:

### Online

When applying online at www.va.gov/healthbenefits/enroll Veterans simply fill out the application and electronically submit it to VA for processing. No need to submit additional documents with your application to verify your military service. VA will search for your supporting military information through our electronic information systems and will contact you if VA is unable to locate your information. For help filling out the application, call 1-877-222-VETS (8387) between 8AM and 8PM ET, Monday - Friday, or click on the "chat online with representative" button located on the website and a representative will provide assistance.

### By Mail

The application form can be downloaded from www.va.gov/healthbenefits/enroll. Complete the form and mail it to:

Health Eligibility Center
Enrollment Eligibility Division
2957 Clairmont Road Suite 200
Atlanta, GA 30329-1647

### By Phone

If you prefer to complete the application over the phone, or have a paper copy mailed to you, you may do so by calling 1-877-222-VETS (8387) between 8AM and 8PM ET, Monday - Friday.

### In Person

You may also apply in person at any VA health care facility.

### You Select Where You Want to Receive Your Care

As part of the enrollment process, Veterans will be given the opportunity to select the VA health care facility or Community Based Outpatient Clinic (CBOC) to serve as his or her preferred facility. To find a facility near you, visit VA's directory at www.va.gov/directory.

## Non-VA Provider Health Care

Many enrolled Veterans now have the option to receive care by a non-VA health care provider closer to home rather than waiting for a VA appointment or traveling long distance to a VA facility. The VA Choice Program temporarily authorizes enrolled Veterans to receive health care from non-VA providers. The following conditions apply:

- Veteran must be enrolled as of August 1, 2014, or is a combat Veteran who served on active duty in a theater of combat operations during a period of war after the Persian Gulf War, or in combat against a hostile force, and is within 5 years of separation. Combat Veterans who were discharged between January 2009 and January 2011, and did not enroll in the VA health care during their 5 year period of eligibility have an additional one year to enroll and receive care. The additional one-year eligibility period began February 12, 2015, with the signing of the Clay Hunt Suicide Prevention for America Veterans Act.

- Wait times for VA care exceed 30 days from the desired care date or the date medically determined by your physician.

- The non-VA care is prescribed by a VA provider.

- Veteran's home is more than 40 miles from to the nearest VA care site – VAMC, community-based outpatient clinic (CBOC), etc.

- Veteran's home is less than 40 miles from a VA medical facility, but must travel by air, boat, or ferry to reach such a facility.

- Veteran resides less than 40 miles from a VA medical facility, but face an unusual or excessive burden in getting to that facility because of geographical challenges.

- Veteran resides in a state without full-service VA medical facilities that provides hospital care, emergency service and surgical care and reside more than 20 miles from such facility.

Non-VA care is only covered by VA for medical needs that have been approved by a VA physician. Enrolled Veterans were mailed a letter and a Choice Card containing details about the program. Veterans who choose to use their Choice Card should coordinate pre-approved care by calling 1-866-606-8198.

Marine Veteran Sgt. Robert "Strong Leg Bull" Norman prepares to push off the wall for the backstroke during swimming practice for the 2012 Warrior Games at Colorado Springs, Colo., April 24. Photo by Lance Cpl. Daniel Wetzel/Flickr

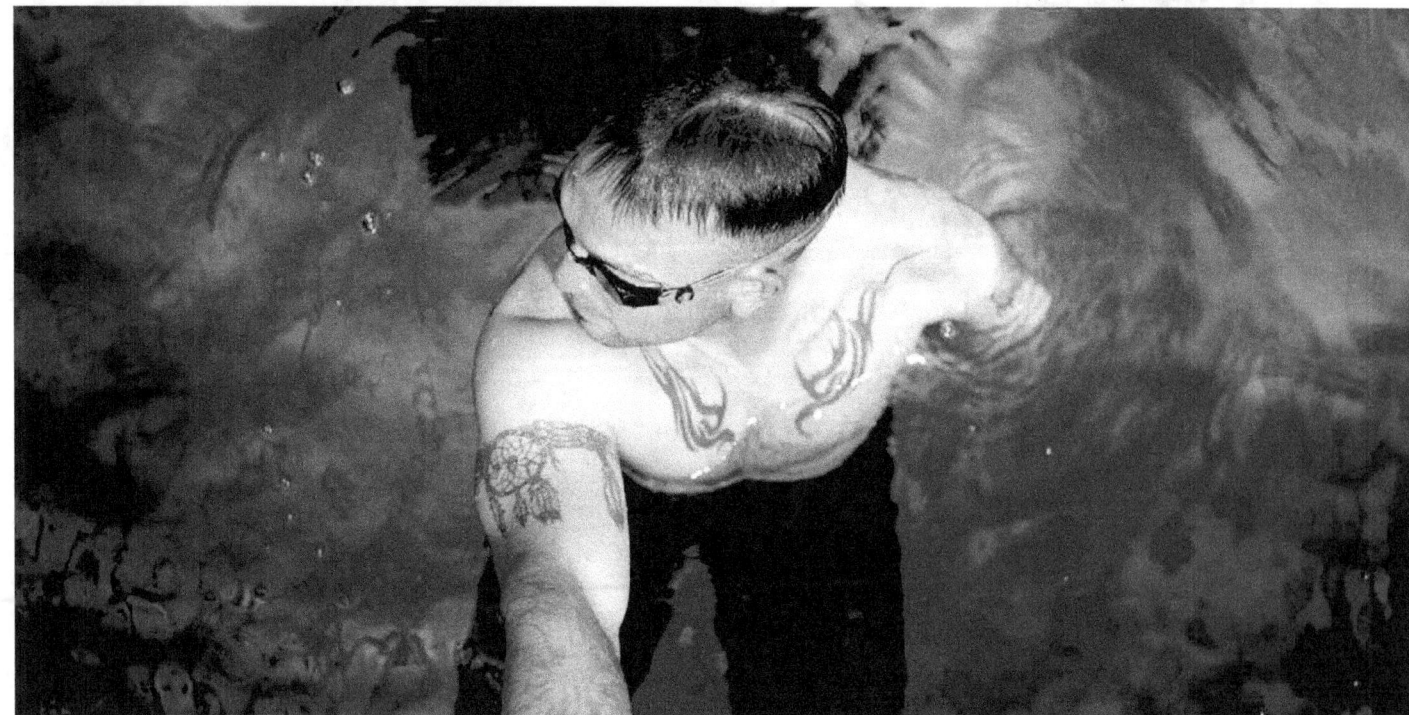

## Enrollment Priority Groups - What are they and how does it work?

The number of Veterans who can be enrolled in the health care program is determined by the amount of money Congress gives VA each year. Since funds are limited, VA set up Priority Groups to make sure that certain groups of Veterans are able to be enrolled before others.

Once you apply for enrollment, your eligibility will be determined based on your specific eligibility information. You will then be assigned a Priority Group based on your specific eligibility. The Priority Groups range from 1-8 with 1 being the highest priority for enrollment. Some high-income Veterans who do not have a special eligibility factor such as a Purple Heart or Medal of Honor for example, may have to agree to pay copays to be placed in certain Priority Groups and may not be eligible for enrollment.

You may be eligible for more than one Enrollment Priority Group. In that case, VA will always place you in the highest Priority Group for which you are eligible.

## Priority Groups

**Priority Group 1**

- Veterans with VA-rated service-connected disabilities 50% or more disabling.
- Veterans determined by VA to be unemployable due to service-connected conditions.

**Priority Group 2**

- Veterans with VA-rated service-connected disabilities 30% or 40% disabling.

**Priority Group 3**

- Veterans who are Former Prisoners of War (POWs).
- Veterans awarded a Purple Heart medal.
- Veterans whose discharge was for a disability that was incurred or aggravated in the line of duty.
- Veterans with VA-rated service-connected disabilities 10% or 20% disabling.
- Veterans awarded special eligibility classification under Title 38, U.S.C., § 1151, "benefits for individuals disabled by treatment or vocational rehabilitation".
- Veterans awarded the Medal of Honor (MOH).

**Priority Group 4**

- Veterans who are receiving aid and attendance or housebound benefits from VA.
- Veterans who have been determined by VA to be catastrophically disabled.

**Priority Group 5**

- Nonservice-connected Veterans and noncompensable service-connected Veterans rated 0% disabled by VA with annual income and/or net worth below the VA income limit and geographically-adjusted income limit for their resident location.
- Veterans receiving VA pension benefits.
- Veterans eligible for Medicaid programs.

**Priority Group 6**

- Compensable 0% service-connected Veterans.
- Veterans exposed to Ionizing Radiation during atmospheric testing or during the occupation of Hiroshima and Nagasaki.
- Project 112/SHAD participants.

- Veterans who served in the Republic of Vietnam between January 9, 1962 and May 7, 1975.
- Veterans of the Persian Gulf War who served in the Southwest Asia Theater of combat operations between August 2, 1990, and November 11, 1998.
- Veterans who served on active duty at Camp Lejeune for not fewer than 30 days beginning August 1, 1953 and ending December 31, 1987*.
- Veterans who served in a theater of combat operations after November 11, 1998, as follows:
  - Currently enrolled Veterans and new enrollees who were discharged from active duty on or after January 28, 2003, are eligible for the enhanced benefits for 5 years post discharge.
  - Combat Veterans who were discharged between January 2009 and January 2011, and did not enroll in the VA health care during their 5 year period of eligibility have an additional one year to enroll and receive care. The additional one-year eligibility period began February 12, 2015 with the signing of the Clay Hunt Suicide Prevention for America Veterans Act.

**Note:** At the end of this enhanced enrollment priority group placement time period, Veterans will be assigned to the highest Priority Group their unique eligibility status at that time qualifies for.

*While eligible for Priority Group (PG) 6; until system changes are implemented you would be assigned to PG 7 or 8 depending on your income.

**Priority Group 7**

- Veterans with gross household income below the geographically-adjusted VA income limit for their resident location and who agree to pay copays.

**Priority Group 8**

- Veterans with gross household incomes above the VA income limits and the geographically-adjusted income limits for their resident location and who agrees to pay copays.

**Veterans eligible for enrollment:** Noncompensable 0% service-connected and:

- **Subpriority a:** Enrolled as of January 16, 2003, and who have remained enrolled since that date and/or placed in this subpriority due to changed eligibility status.
- **Subpriority b:** Enrolled on or after June 15, 2009, whose income exceeds the current VA income limits or the geographically-adjusted VA income limits by 10% or less.

**Veterans eligible for enrollment:** Nonservice-connected and:

- **Subpriority c:** Enrolled as of January 16, 2003, and who have remained enrolled since that date and/or placed in this subpriority due to changed eligibility status.
- **Subpriority d:** Enrolled on or after June 15, 2009, whose income exceeds the current VA income limit and geographic income limit by 10% or less.

**Veterans not eligible for enrollment:** Veterans not meeting the criteria above:

- **Subpriority e:** Noncompensable 0% service-connected (eligible for care of their SC condition only).
- **Subpriority g:** Nonservice-connected.

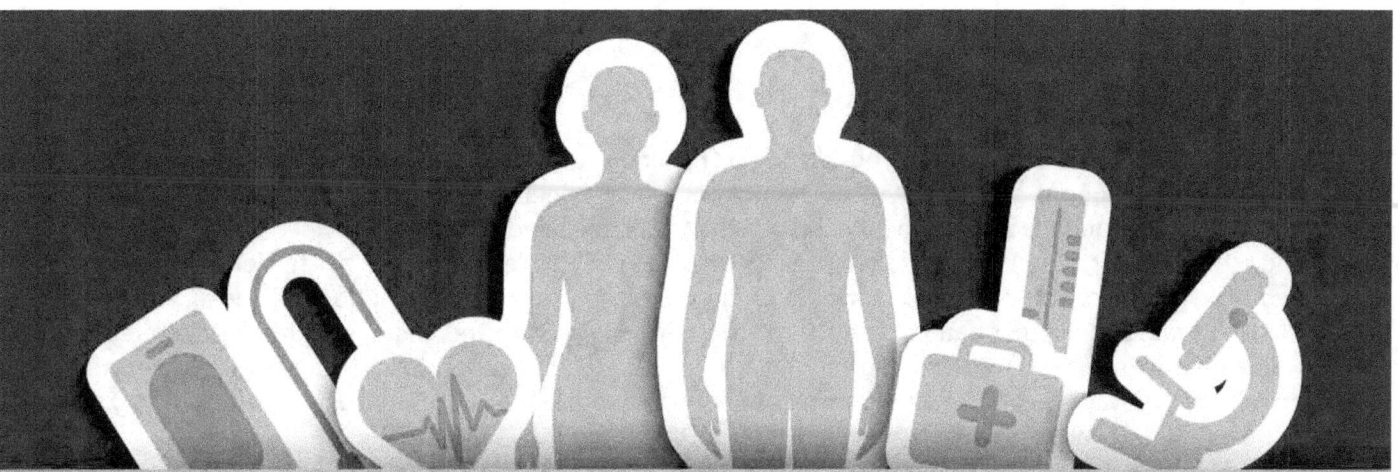

# What is Quality Care?

"Quality care" has many definitions, but at VA it means:

- The right type of care for your health condition
- Care that results in the best possible outcome for you
- Care delivered with attention to your concerns, needs, and life goals
- Care that keeps you safe from hazards and harm

**Visit VA's Quality of Care site at
www.va.gov/qualityofcare/ to see how
we are doing!**

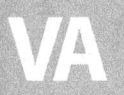 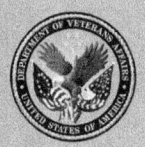 **U.S. Department of Veterans Affairs**
Veterans Health Administration

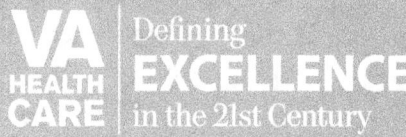

## Once Enrolled

Once your enrollment is confirmed, you can begin enjoying your VA health care benefits. You will receive a welcoming telephone call from VA staff. During that call, we can answer many of your initial questions and share information regarding your health benefits and other various services provided through VA, and schedule your initial VA health care appointment. You will also receive a personalized letter and a Veterans Health Benefits handbook in the mail within 10 business days. The handbook will detail your VA health care benefit information, based on your specific eligibility factors, in an organized, easy-to-read format. It also includes information on your preferred facility, copay responsibilities, how to schedule appointments, ways to communicate treatment needs, and more. For more information, visit www.va.gov/HEALTHBENEFITS/vhbh/index.asp.

## Keep your Personal Information Updated

While you are enrolled, you can update or report changes to your address, phone number, name, health insurance or financial information by completing VA Form 10-10EZR Health Benefits Renewal Form on-line at www.va.gov/healthbenefits. By keeping your information updated, it allows VA to better inform you of updates to benefits and services. You may also call VA's toll-free number at 1-877-222-VETS (8387) between 8AM and 8PM ET, Monday – Friday, or contact the Enrollment Coordinator at your local medical facility. You may also use the self-service kiosks available at most VA Health care facilities to update your personal information. See page 36 for more information about the kiosks.

## Your Information is secure with the Veteran Health Identification Card

VA issues enrolled Veterans a Veteran Health Identification Card (VHIC) for use at VA health care facilities. The VHIC safeguards your personal information – the Member ID and Card Number have eliminated the need for your Social Security number to be on the card. Similar to a typical health insurance card, the VHIC signifies your enrollment in VA health care.

The VHIC is used as proof of identity, and to check in for appointments at VA health care facilities. While the card is not required to receive health care, VA recommends all enrolled Veterans obtain a card.

To obtain a VHIC, you will need to provide two forms of identification, such as your driver's license or passport to your local VA health care facility and have your photo taken. The card will be mailed to you, usually within 7 to 10 days after the card has been requested. For more information about the types of identification needed go to page 47. You may also visit www.va.gov/healthbenefits/vhic, or call 1-877-222-VETS (8387) between 8AM and 8PM ET, Monday - Friday.

## Schedule an Appointment

You may request a doctor's appointment at the time you apply for enrollment. An appointment will be made with a VA doctor or provider and you will be notified via mail of the appointment date and time. If you need health care before your scheduled appointment, you may contact the Enrollment Coordinator, Urgent Care Clinic or the Emergency Room at your local VA medical facility.

## You Will Be Assigned A Personalized Care Team

Today, Veterans will experience primary care at VA very differently than they did five years ago. Every patient is assigned a health care team they can count on to help coordinate and personalize their care. Every Patient Aligned Care Team (PACT) includes a primary care provider, clinical pharmacist, RN care manager, LPN or medical assistant and clerk. A Veteran can expect their PACT to help them use health care services, including eHealth technologies, which are necessary to optimize their health and well-being. For more information, visit: www.va.gov/health/services/primarycare/pact or visit the Enrollment Coordinator at the local VA medical facility.

## Financial Reporting Requirements

While many Veterans qualify for enrollment and cost-free health care services based on a compensable service-connected condition or other qualifying factors, certain Veterans will be asked to complete a financial assessment at the time of enrollment to determine their eligibility for cost-free medical care, medications and/or travel benefits. The assessment is based on the Veteran's, (spouse and dependents, if any) previous year gross household income. This financial information may also be used to determine the Veteran's enrollment priority group. For more information, visit www.va.gov/HEALTHBENEFITS/cost/financial_assessment.asp, call VA's toll-free number at 1-877-222-VETS (8387) between 8AM and 8PM ET, Monday – Friday, or contact the Enrollment Coordinator at the local VA medical facility.

***Note:*** VA eliminated the annual requirement for updated financial information. VA now uses information from the Internal Revenue Service and Social Security Administration to automatically match individual Veterans' income information, which reduces the burden on Veterans to keep their healthcare eligibility up to date.

## Net Worth Information No Longer Required

Effective January 2015, VA eliminated the use of net worth information as a determining factor for eligibility in both medical care services and copayment responsibilities. This change makes VA health care benefits more accessible to lower-income Veterans, who have no service-connected condition or other qualifying factors. VA will now only consider a Veteran's gross household income and deductible expenses from the previous year.

At the Union pier in downtown Charleston, Coast Guard Cutter Hamilton crew rehearse for the Cutter Hamilton's upcoming commissioning ceremony Dec. 4, 2014.                     U.S. Coast Guard photo by Senior Chief Petty Officer Sarah B. Foster/ Flickr

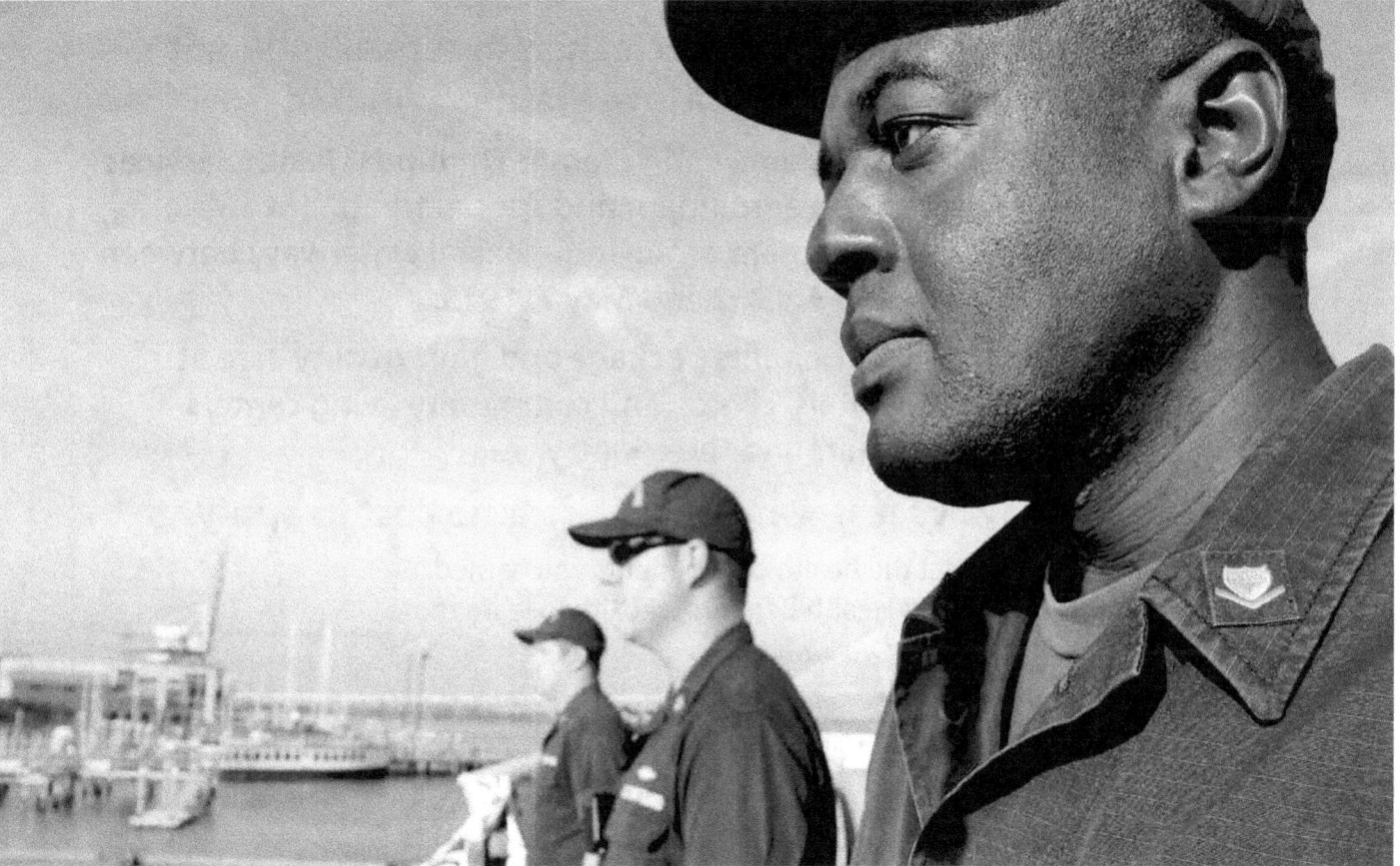

### Use Our Online Tool to Determine Your Eligibility Based on Income

Our Financial Calculator at hbexplorer.vacloud.us can be used to help determine whether your income would be considered in determining your enrollment eligibility.

If you are denied enrollment because your household income exceeds the income limit, VA's Financial Hardship program could help qualify you for enrollment if you have had a recent change in your income, such as a loss of employment. For more information, refer to the Financial Hardship Section on page 14.

VA income limit information can be found online at nationalincomelimits.vaftl.us.

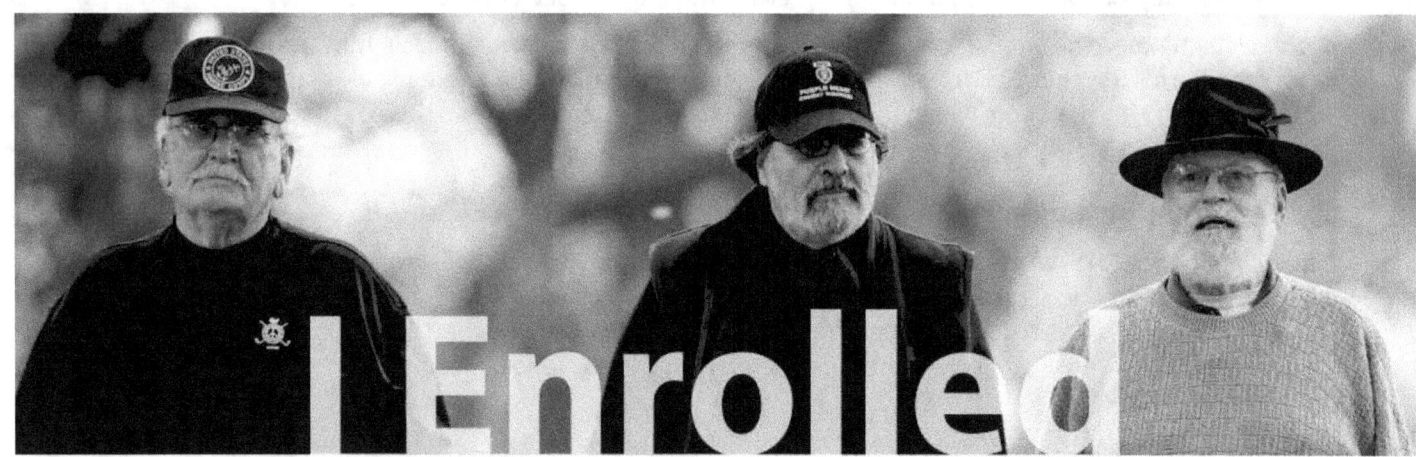

## "I Served in Vietnam. Now I'm taking advantage of the health benefits I have earned."

### Did you know VA provides special health care enrollment opportunities and benefits to Vietnam Veterans?

**Public Law 111-163, the Caregivers and Veterans Omnibus Health Services Act of 2012 reestablished VA's enrollment and special treatment authority for Veterans who served in Vietnam or the intracoastal waterways between January 9, 1962 and May 7, 1975.**

**VA offers a full medical benefits package and high-quality care at more than 1,700 hospitals, clinics, and community living centers around the country.**

### Enroll today. It's fast, easy and there is no cost to apply.

Get the health care benefits you earned.
Visit VA's Health Benefits website to learn more.
www.va.gov/healthbenefits

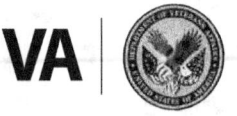

**U.S. Department of Veterans Affairs**

Veterans Health Administration
*Chief Business Office*
*Health Eligibility Center*

# Copayments

## Types of Copayments

 **No copayments are charged for treatment of service-connected conditions.**

### Outpatient Copayments*

—based on the highest of two levels of service on any individual day.

- **Primary Care Services** – Services provided in a primary care setting to address overall patient care
- **Specialty Care Services** – Services provided in Specialty Care area such as:
  - Surgery
  - Radiology
  - Audiology
  - Optometry
  - Cardiology
  - and specialty tests such as:
    - magnetic resonance imagery (MRI)
    - computerized axial tomography (CAT) scan
    - nuclear medicine studies (highest level of service)

*There is no copay requirement for preventive care services such as screenings or immunizations.*

### Medication Copayments*

— applicable to each prescription, including each 30-day supply or less of maintenance medications.

*Includes an annual cap for enrollment priority groups 2 through 6.*

### Inpatient Copayments

— in addition to a standard copay charge for each 90 days of care within a 365 day period regardless of the level of service (such as intensive care, surgical care or general medical care); a per diem (daily) charge will be assessed for each day of hospitalization.

### Long-Term Care Copayments*

— based on three levels of care (see Long-Term Care Benefits on page 22 for definitions).

- Community Living Centers (Nursing Home) Care/Inpatient Respite Care/Geriatric Evaluation
- Adult Day Health Care/Outpatient Geriatric Evaluation/Outpatient Respite Care
- Domiciliary Care

*Copayments for Long-Term Care services start on the 22nd day of care during any 12-month period — there is no copay requirement for the first 21 days. Actual copay charges will vary from Veteran to Veteran depending on financial information submitted on VA Form 10-10EC.*

**NOTE:** There are no copayments for hospice care provided in any setting.

## Outpatient Copayments

- **Primary Care Services** – services provided by a primary care clinician – $15
- **Specialty Care Services** – In general, services delivered in a specialty outpatient clinic provided by highly- specialized, narrowly-focused health care professionals-services provided by a clinical specialist– Specialty Copay – $50

## Inpatient Copayments

There are two inpatient copay rates – the full rate and the reduced rate. The reduced inpatient copay rate, which is 20% of the full inpatient rate, applies to Veterans enrolled in Priority Group 7. Both the full inpatient copay rate and the reduced inpatient copay rate are computed over a 365 - day period. Because the Inpatient Copay rates change each year, they are published separately and can be found on line at www.va.gov/healthbenefits/cost or for more information, contact VA at 1-877-222-VETS (8387) between 8AM and 8PM ET, Monday - Friday.

## Medication Copayments

Currently, there is a $8 copay (subject to change) for each 30-day or less supply of medication provided on an outpatient basis for treatment of a nonservice-connected condition for Veterans in Priority Group 2 through 6, with an annual copayment cap of $960, unless otherwise exempted. This copay is $9 for Veterans in Priority Group 7 or 8 with no annual copayment cap.

Even though a prescription may be written for 90 days, each 30-day or less supply is subject to that year's applicable medication copay rate. A 90-day supply would cost three times the applicable medication copay rate based on your Priority Group.

## Long Term Care Copayments

Long term care copay are based on three levels of care

- **Inpatient:** Up to $97 per day (Nursing Home, Respite, Geriatric Evaluation)
- **Outpatient:** $15 per day (Adult Day Health Care, Respite, Geriatric Evaluation)
- **Domiciliary:** $5 per day

## Annual Changes to Copay Rates

Copay rates may change annually — including the annual cap on medication copayments. Current year rates can be obtained at any VA health care facility or on VA's web site at www.va.gov/healthbenefits/cost/copay_rates.asp.

## Veterans Not Required to Make Copayments

Many Veterans qualify for cost-free health care and/or medications based on:

- Receipt of a Purple Heart, or
- Medal of Honor, or
- Former Prisoner of War Status, or
- 50% or more Compensable VA service-connected disabilities, (0-40% service-connected may take co-pay test to determine medication copay status), or
- Veterans deemed catastrophically disabled by a VA provider, or
- Veterans with income below the income limit, or
- Other qualifying factors, including treatment related to their military service experience.

## Services Exempt from Inpatient and Outpatient Copayments

*(Partial list)*

- Special registry examinations offered by VA to evaluate possible health risks associated with military service
- Counseling and care for military sexual trauma
- Compensation and pension examinations are requested by the Veterans Benefits Administration (VBA).

This is a physical exam to determine service-related illness or injuries for determination of a Veteran's entitlement to compensation and pension benefits.

- Care that is part of a VA-approved research project
- Care related to a VA-rated service-connected disability
- Readjustment counseling and related mental health services
- Care for cancer of head or neck caused by nose or throat radium treatments received while in the military
- Catastrophic disability exam
- Individual or group smoking cessation or weight reduction services
- Publicly announced VA public health initiatives, for example, health fairs
- Care potentially related to combat service for Veterans that served in a theater of combat operations after November 11, 1998. This benefit is effective for 5 years after the date of Veteran's most recent discharge from active duty. Combat Veterans who were discharged between January 2009 and January 2011, and did not enroll in the VA health care during their 5 year period of eligibility have an additional one year to enroll and receive care. The additional one-year eligibility period began February 12, 2015, with the signing of the Clay Hunt Suicide Prevention for America Veterans Act.
- Laboratory and electrocardiograms

# Struggling To Pay VA Copayments? VA Has Programs That Can Help

VA has programs that can assist enrolled Veterans who may be suffering from financial distress, struggling to pay VA copayments, lost a job or currently face a significant decrease in household income. VA's medical care hardship program could help Veterans qualify for VA health care enrollment for health care services if they had a recent change in their income, even if they were previously denied enrollment based on their household income. Veterans who have not applied for VA enrollment because they thought their income was too high may want to reconsider applying if their projected current year's income is lower. Personal circumstances, such as loss of employment, sudden decrease in income or increases in out-of- pocket Veteran or family health care expenses, can all be reasons for VA to consider a Veteran's financial hardship.

| Four possible options for Veterans unable to pay assessed copay charges | |
| --- | --- |
| Hardship Determination | A Hardship Determination provides an exemption from outpatient and inpatient copays for the remaining calendar year. If your projected household income is substantially below your prior year's income, you may request a Hardship Determination by contacting your local Enrollment Coordinator. |
| Waiver | A waiver or "write-off" refers to an agreement to forgive payment of an existing VA debt. If your projected household income for the current year is substantially reduced and will affect your ability to repay your debt, you can request a waiver of your copayment debt. You must request a waiver within 180 days of the date of your billing statement. To request a waiver, contact your local Revenue Office or call VA at 1-877-222-VETS (8387). |
| Offer in Compromise | A compromise is an "offer to settle" your past VA debts. VA will consider both current and future household income in making a determination. Generally, offers of compromise that are accepted must be paid in full within 30 days from the date of acceptance.<br><br>**To request a compromise, contact your local Revenue Office.** |
| Repayment Plans | Another option that may be available to you is a VA repayment plan, known as "collection by installment." To request a repayment plan, contact your local Revenue Office or call VA at 1-877-222-VETS (8387) between 8AM and 8PM ET, Monday – Friday. |

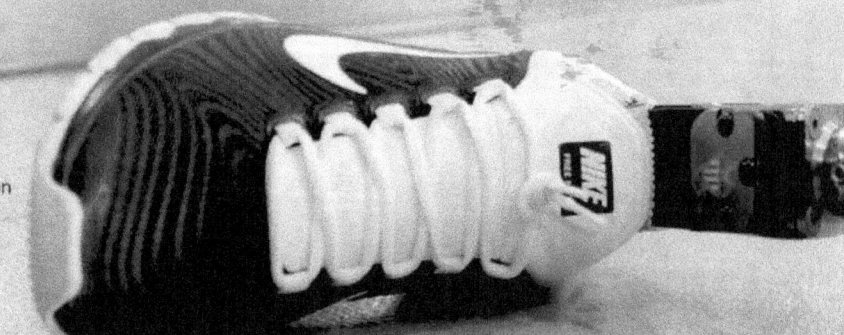

A prosthetic leg sits beside the volleyball court as the U.S. Invictus Games seated volleyball team practices for competition. Invictus Games is an international competition that brings together wounded, injured and ill service members in the spirit of friendly athletic competition. (U.S. Navy photo by Mass Communication Specialist 2nd Class Joshua D. Sheppard/Released)

## VA's Medical Care Hardship program may help you qualify for VA Health Care enrollment

If your income has recently changed, you may qualify for enrollment even if it was denied previously based on your household income. Or, perhaps you have put off applying for enrollment because you think your income is too high. Now may be the time to provide updated financial information or apply for enrollment.

Personal circumstances, such as loss of employment, sudden decrease in income, or increases of out-of-pocket family health care expenses factor into VA's hardship determination.

If your current and projected household income puts you below the VA Income Limits or Geographic Income Limits for your area, you may qualify for enrollment and cost-free VA medical care.

For more information and qualifications for this program, contact your local VA at 1-877-222 VETS (8387) between 8AM and 8PM ET, Monday – Friday.

## Veterans with Catastrophic Disabilities

VA provides special enrollment considerations for Veterans with a Catastrophic Disability. To be considered catastrophically disabled, a Veteran must be determined by a VA provider to have a severely disabling injury, disorder or disease that compromises their ability to carry out the activities of daily living to such a degree that personal or mechanical assistance is required to leave home or bed, or constant supervision is required to avoid physical harm to themselves or others.

Veterans may request a catastrophic disability evaluation by contacting the Enrollment Coordinator at their local VA health care facility. VA will make every effort to schedule an evaluation within 30 days of the request, and there is no charge for the Catastrophic Disability evaluation. If found to be catastrophically disabled, the Veteran will be enrolled and receive cost- free care for outpatient and inpatient VA medical care and medications; however, Veterans in this category may be subject to copayments for extended care (long-term care).

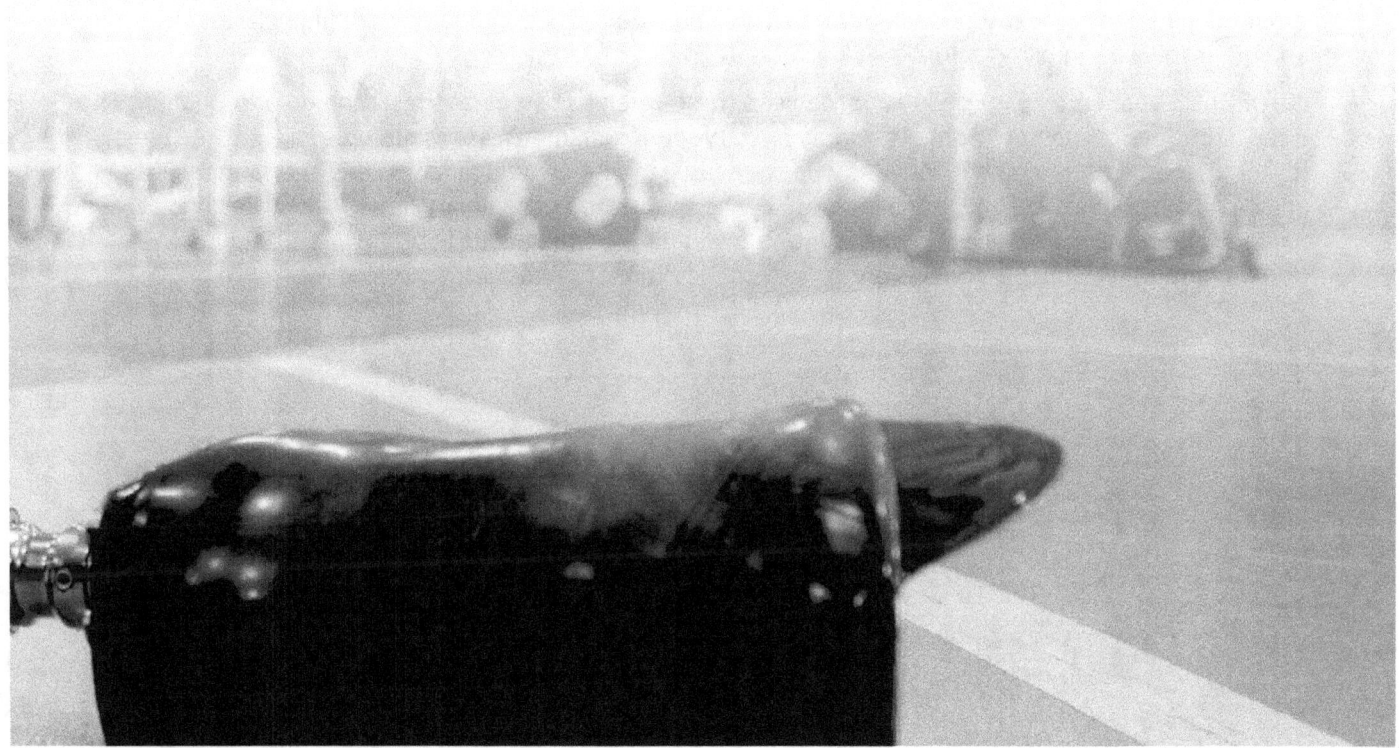

# Basic Eligibility for VA Health Care

If you served in the active military, naval or air service and are separated under any condition other than dishonorable, you may qualify for VA health care benefits. Current and former members of the Reserves or National Guard who were called to active duty (other than for training only) by a federal order and completed the full period for which they were called or ordered to active duty may be eligible for VA health care as well.

## Minimum Duty Requirements

Most Veterans who enlisted after September 7, 1980, or entered active duty after October 16, 1981, must have served 24 continuous months or the full period for which they were called to active duty to be eligible. This minimum duty requirement may not apply to Veterans who were discharged for a disability incurred or aggravated in the line of duty, discharged for a hardship, or received an "early out." Since there are a number of other exceptions to the minimum duty requirements, VA encourages all Veterans to apply to determine their enrollment eligibility.

### Returning Service Members (OEF/OIF/OND)

Every VA medical center has a team ready to welcome OEF/OIF/OND Service members, and to help coordinate their health care and other services. For more information about the various programs available for recent returning Service members, log on to the Returning Service members web site at www.oefoif.va.gov.

Veterans who served in a theater of operations also have special eligibility for VA health care. Under the "Combat Veteran" authority VA provides cost-free health care services and nursing home care for conditions possibly related to military service and enrollment in Priority Group 6 or higher for 5 years from the date of discharge or release from active duty, unless eligible for enrollment in a higher priority group.

Combat Veterans who enroll with VA under this enhanced Combat Veteran authority will continue to be enrolled even after their enhanced eligibility period ends, although they may be shifted to a lower Priority Group, depending on their income level, and required to make applicable copayments. Additionally, for care not related to combat service, copayments may be required depending on their financial assessment and other special eligibility factors.

**NOTE:** The 5-year enrollment period applicable to these Veterans begins on the discharge or separation date of the Service member from active duty military service, or in the case of multiple call-ups, the most recent discharge date. Combat Veterans who were discharged between January 2009 and January 2011, and did not enroll in the VA health care during their 5 year period of eligibility have an additional one year to enroll and receive care. The additional one-year eligibility period began February 12, 2015, with the signing of the Clay Hunt Suicide Prevention for America Veterans Act.

# You Are Covered Under The Affordable Care Act

The Affordable Care Act, also known as the health care law, was created to expand access to coverage, control health care costs and improve health care quality and care coordination. The health care law does not change VA health benefits or Veterans' out-of-pocket costs.

Three things you should know:

1. VA wants all Veterans to receive health care that improves their health and well-being.

2. If you are enrolled in any of VA's programs below, you have coverage under the standards of the health care law:

   - Veteran's health care program
   - Civilian Health and Medical program (CHAMPVA)
   - Spina bifida health care program

3. If you are not enrolled in VA health care, you can apply at any time.

Your family members who are not enrolled in a VA health care program and who do not meet the health care law coverage standards should use the Marketplace to get coverage. The Marketplace remains available during non-Open Season periods for individuals who have a qualifying life event, such as getting married or having a baby. For more information about the Marketplace, visit www.healthcare.gov or call 1-800-318-2596.

*Note:* U.S. taxpayers will need to declare that they have health coverage on their federal tax forms. There's no specific forms, just check "Full-year coverage" on Line 61 on Internal Revenue Service Form 1040, Line 38 on the 1040A , and various other entries on IRS income tax forms. Starting in 2016, VA will send IRS, Veterans and eligible beneficiaries forms that provide details of the health coverage provided by VA. These forms are to be used for the income tax process. For more information about ACA and VA health care, visit VA's website at www.va.gov/aca or call 1-877-222-VETS (8387) Monday - Friday between 8 AM and 8 PM ET.

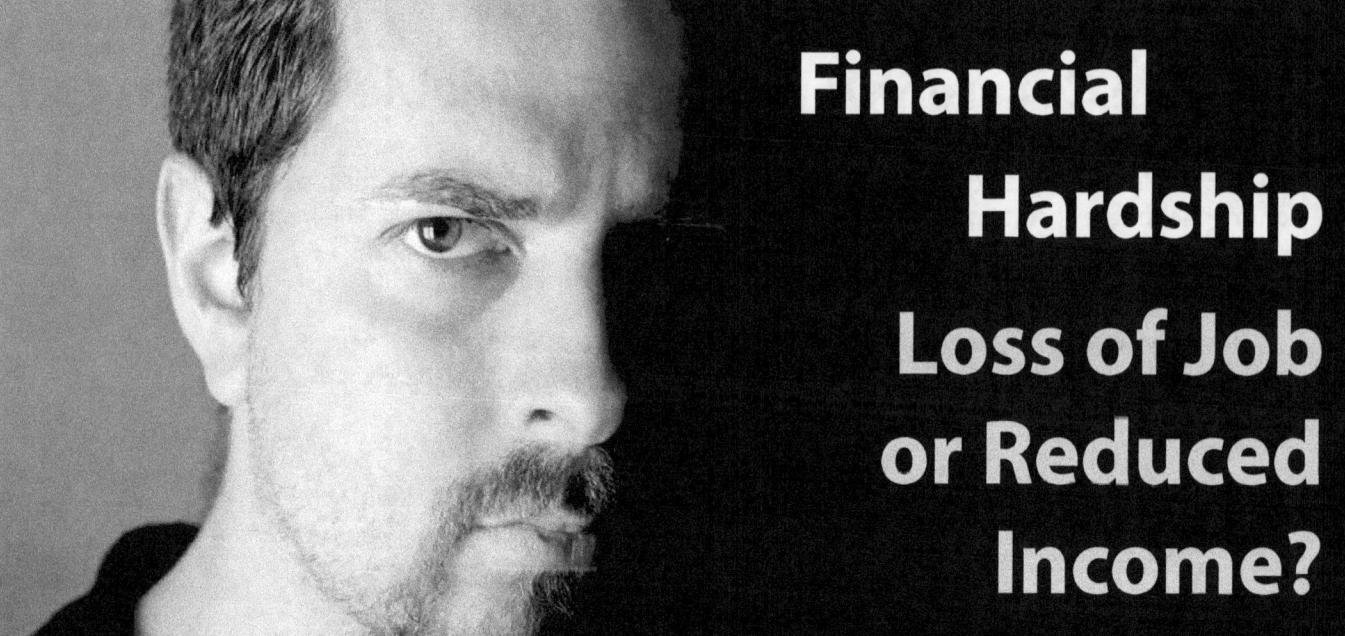

# Financial Hardship

# Loss of Job or Reduced Income?

## VA's Medical Care Hardship program may help you qualify for VA Health Care enrollment

If your income has recently changed, you may qualify for enrollment even if it was denied previously based on your household income. Or, perhaps you have put off applying for enrollment because you think your income is too high. Now may be the time to provide updated financial information or apply for enrollment.

Personal circumstances such as loss of employment, sudden decrease in income, or increases of out-of-pocket family health care expenses factor into VA's hardship determination.

If your current and projected household income puts you below the VA income limits or geographic income limits for your area, you may qualify for enrollment and cost-free VA medical care.

For additional information and qualifications for this program, contact your local VA Medical Center Enrollment Coordinator at:

**1-877-222 VETS (8387)**

For more information, call toll-free
1-877-222 VETS (8387) or visit our website at
www.va.gov/healthbenefits/

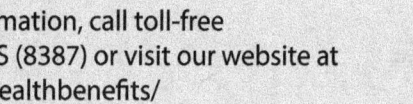 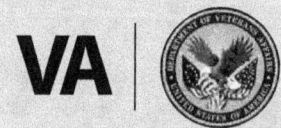

**U.S. Department of Veterans Affairs**
Veterans Health Administration
Chief Business Office
Health Eligibility Center

# VA and Other Health Insurance

If you have other forms of health care coverage, such as a private insurance plan, Medicare, Medicaid or TRICARE, you can continue to use VA along with these plans. Remember: it is always a good idea to inform your doctors if you are receiving care outside of VA, so your health care can be coordinated.

## Private Health Insurance

Veterans with private health insurance may choose to use these sources of coverage as a supplement to their VA benefits. Also, Veterans are not responsible for payment of VA medical services billed to their health insurance company that are not paid by their insurance carrier.

By law, VA is obligated to bill health insurance carriers for services provided to treat a Veteran's nonservice-connected conditions. Veterans are asked to disclose all relevant health insurance information to ensure current insurance information is on file—including coverage through a spouse. Identification of insurance information is essential to VA because collections received from private health insurance companies help supplement the funding available to provide services to additional Veterans. Enrolled Veterans may now provide any changes in their insurance by:

- Using the online Health Benefits Renewal (10-10-EZR) form at https://www.1010ez.med.va.gov/ or
- Calling 1-877-222-VETS (8387) Monday - Friday between 8 AM and 8 PM ET, or
- Using the self-service touch Kiosks available at their local VA health care facility.

It is important to note that VA health care is NOT considered a health insurance plan.

### *CAUTION!*

Before canceling health insurance coverage, enrolled Veterans should carefully consider the risks.

- There is no guarantee that in subsequent years Congress will appropriate sufficient funds for VA to provide care for all enrollment priority groups.
- Non-Veteran spouses and other family members generally do not qualify for VA health care.
- If participation in Medicare Part B is cancelled, it cannot be reinstated until January of the next year, and there may be a penalty for the reinstatement.
- Provides additional coverage for Veterans who receive care from VA and non-VA providers.

# Medicare Part D Prescription Drug Coverage

## Creditable Coverage

If you are eligible for Medicare Part D prescription drug coverage, you need to know that enrollment in the VA health care system is considered creditable coverage for Medicare Part D purposes. This means that VA prescription drug coverage is at least as good as the Medicare Part D coverage. Since only Veterans may enroll in the VA health care system, dependents and family members do not receive credible coverage under the Veteran's enrollment.

However, there is one significant area in which VA health care is NOT creditable coverage: Medicare Part B (outpatient health care, including doctors' fees). Creditable coverage for Medicare Part B can only be provided through an **employer**. As a result, VA health care benefits to Veterans are not creditable coverage for the Part B program. So although a Veteran may avoid the late enrollment penalty for Medicare Part D by citing VA health care enrollment, that enrollment would not help the Veteran avoid the late enrollment penalty for Part B.

VA does not recommend Veterans cancel or decline coverage in Medicare (or other health care or insurance programs) solely because they are enrolled in VA health care. Unlike Medicare, which offers the same benefits for all enrollees, VA assigns enrollees to enrollment priority groups, based on a variety of eligibility factors, such as service-connection and income. There is no guarantee that in subsequent years Congress will appropriate sufficient medical care funds for VA to provide care for all enrollment priority groups. This could leave Veterans, especially those enrolled in one of the lower-priority groups, with no access to VA health care coverage. For this reason, having a secondary source of coverage may be in the Veteran's best interest.

In addition, a Veteran may want to consider the flexibility afforded by enrolling in both VA and Medicare. For example, Veterans enrolled in both programs would have access to non-VA physicians (under Medicare Part A or Part B) or may obtain prescription drugs not on the VA formulary if prescribed by non-VA physicians and filled at their local retail pharmacies (under Medicare Part D).

Additional information on Medicare Part D prescription drug coverage can be found online at the Health and Human Services Medicare website at www.medicare.gov.

# Medical Benefits Package

Your comprehensive VA Health Benefits package includes all the necessary inpatient hospital care and outpatient services to promote, preserve, or restore your health. VA medical facilities provide a wide range of services including traditional hospital-based services such as surgery, critical care, mental health, orthopedics, pharmacy, radiology and physical therapy.

In addition, most of our medical facilities offer additional medical and surgical specialty services including audiology & speech pathology, dermatology, dental, geriatrics, neurology, oncology, podiatry, prosthetics, urology, and vision care. Some medical centers also offer advanced services such as organ transplants and plastic surgery.

## Preventive Care Services

- Immunizations
- Physical Examinations (including eye and hearing examinations)
- Health Care Assessments
- Screening Tests
- Health Education Programs

## Ambulatory (Outpatient) Diagnostic and Treatment Services

- Primary and Specialty Care
- Surgical (including reconstructive/plastic surgery as a result of disease or trauma)
- Mental Health
- Substance Abuse

## Hospital (Inpatient) Diagnostic and Treatment Services

- Medical
- Surgical (including reconstructive/plastic surgery as a result of disease or trauma)
- Mental Health
- Substance Abuse
- Prescription Drugs (**when prescribed by a VA physician**)

## Meeting Women Veterans' Unique Needs

Our staff delivers the highest quality health care in a setting that ensures privacy, dignity, and sensitivity. Your local VA facility offers a variety of services, including:

- Women's gender-specific health
- Screening and disease prevention Routine gynecologic services

Female Veterans are potentially eligible to receive care provided in the community when authorized by VA. However, the decision to utilize such care is left to the facility providing your care. By law, purchased-care can only be provided when your treating facility cannot provide you the care you require or because of geographical inaccessibility.

Contact your local VA facility's Women Veterans Program Manager for more information on available services, or call **1-855-VA-WOMEN (1-855-829-6636)**.

# Available Long-Term Care Services

The following is a list of standard benefits. For more information on Extended Care Services and Geriatrics, visit www.va.gov/healthbenefits/access/geriatrics.asp.

## VA Community Living Centers (VA Nursing Home) Programs

While some Veterans qualify for indefinite Community Living Center (formerly known as nursing home care) services, other Veterans may qualify for a limited period of time.

## Domiciliary Care

Domiciliary care provides rehabilitative and long-term, health maintenance care for Veterans who require some medical care, but who do not require all the services provided in nursing homes. Domiciliary care emphasizes rehabilitation and return to the community.

## Medical Foster Home

Medical Foster Homes are private homes in which a trained caregiver provides services to a few individuals. Some, but not all, residents are Veterans. VA inspects and approves all Medical Foster Homes. Contact your VA social worker or case manager for further information on Medical Foster Home care.

## State Veterans Homes

State Veterans Homes are facilities that provide nursing home, domiciliary or adult day care. Each State establishes eligibility and admission criteria for its homes. For more information about your State Veterans Home, contact the State Veterans home directly or Social Work Service at your local VA facility.

U.S. Marine Corps Cpl. Chester Nez recieves an American flag at Code Talker Hall, Marine Corps Base Quantico, Va., April 4, 2014. Cpl. Nez is the last of the original 29 Navajo Code Talkers of World War II. (U.S. Marine Corps photo by Cpl. Kathryn K. Bynum/Released)

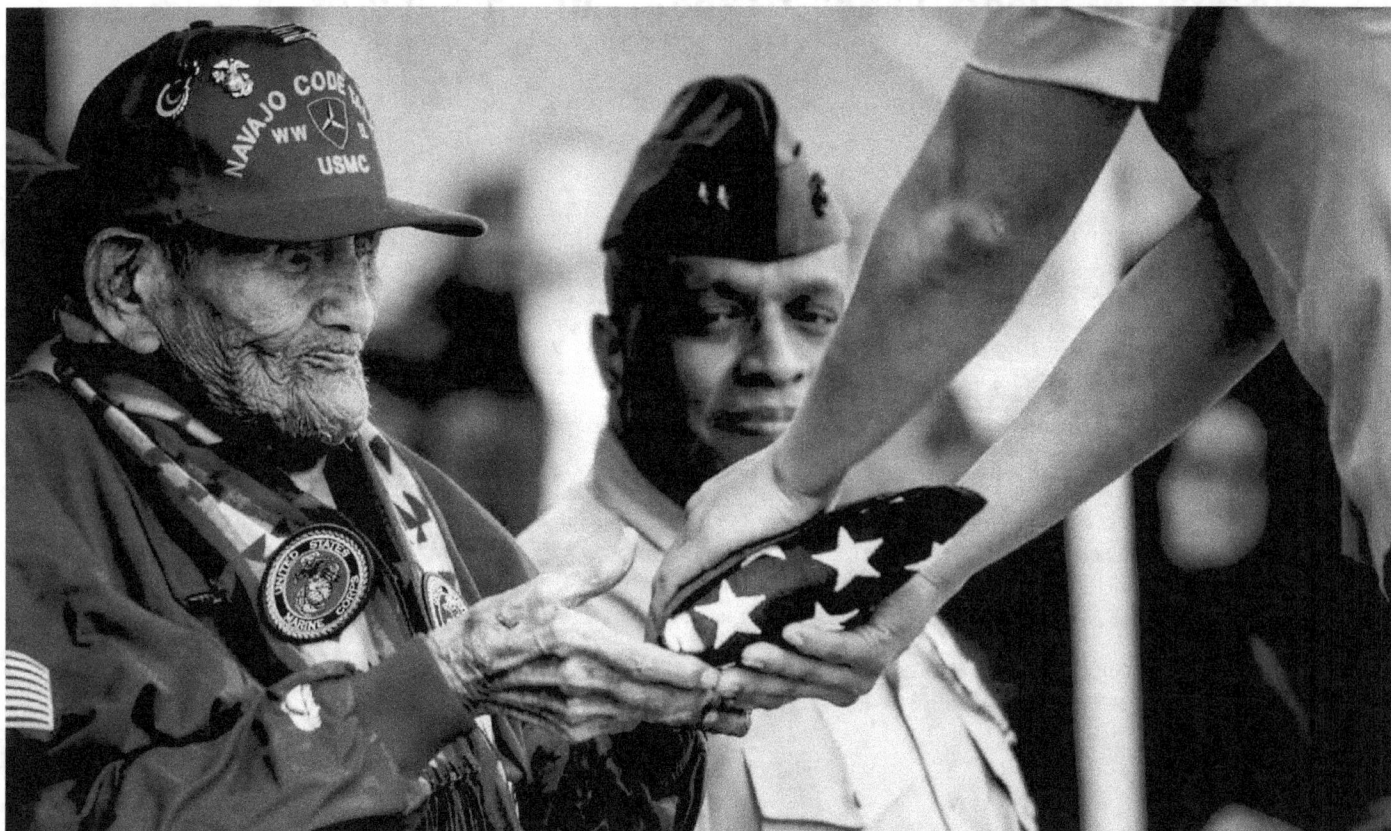

# Additional Services

## Geriatric Evaluation

Geriatric evaluation is the comprehensive assessment of a Veteran's ability to care for him/herself, his/her physical health and social environment, which leads to a plan of care. The plan could include treatment, rehabilitation, health promotion and social services. These evaluations are performed by inpatient Geriatric Evaluation and Management (GEM) Units, GEM clinics, geriatric primary care clinics and other outpatient settings.

## Geriatrics and Extended Care

Geriatrics and Extended Care provides services for Veterans who are elderly and have complex needs, and Veterans of any age who need daily support and assistance. Veterans can receive care at home, at VA medical centers or in the community.

## Adult Day Health Care

Adult Day Health Care is a program Veterans can go to during the day for social activities, peer support, companionship, and recreation. Adult Day Health Care is for Veterans who need skilled services, case management, and assistance with activities of daily living (e.g., bathing and getting dressed) or instrumental activities of daily. Adult Day Health Care can provide respite care for a family caregiver and can also help Veterans and their caregiver gain skills to manage the Veteran's care at home.

## Respite Care

Respite Care is a service that pays for a person to come to a Veteran's home or for a Veteran to go to a program while their family caregiver takes a break. Respite Care services may be available up to 30 days each calendar year.

## Home Health Care

Home Health Care includes VA's Skilled Home Health Care Services (SHHC), Homemaker and Home Health Aide Services (H/HHA) and Family Caregivers Program. For details on these programs, vist www.va.gov/healthbenefits/access/home_health_care.asp.

SHHC is short-term health care services that can be provided to Veterans if they are homebound or live far away from VA. The care is delivered by a community-based home health agency that has a contract with VA.

The services of a Homemaker or Home Health Aide can help Veterans remain living in their own home and can serve Veterans of any age.

VA's Family Caregivers Program provides support and assistance to caregivers of post 9/11 Veterans and Service Members being medically discharged. Eligible primary Family Caregivers can receive a stipend, training, mental health services, travel and lodging reimbursement, and access to health insurance if they are not already under a health care plan. For more information, contact your local VA medical facility and speak with a Caregiver Support Coordinator, visit www.caregiver.va.gov or dial toll-free 1-877-222-VETS (8387) between 8AM and 8PM ET, Monday - Friday.

## Home Telehealth

VA's Home Telehealth, also known as Care Coordination/Home Telehealth, is a service that allows the Veteran's physician or nurse to monitor the Veteran's medical condition remotely using home monitoring equipment. Veterans can be referred to a care coordinator for Home Telehealth services by any member of their care team.

Home Telehealth program aims to make the patient's home the preferred place to receive care, whenever possible.

## Hospice/Palliative Care

Hospice/palliative care is a comfort based form of care for Veterans who have a terminal condition with six months or less to live. Hospice Care provides treatment that relieves suffering and helps to control symptoms in a way that respects your personal, cultural, and religious beliefs and practices. Hospice also provides grief counseling to your family.

**NOTE:** There are no copayments for hospice care provided in any setting.

## Some Veterans receive Free Long-Term Care Services

For Veterans who are not automatically exempt from making copayments for long-term care services (see Copayments on page 11), a separate financial assessment (VA Form 10-10EC, Application for Extended Care Services) must be completed to determine whether they qualify for cost-free services or to what extent they are required to make long-term care copayments. Unlike copayments for other VA health care services, which are based on fixed charges for all, long-term care, copay charges are individually adjusted based on each Veteran's financial status.

## Benefits with Special Eligibility Criteria

While all enrolled Veterans enjoy access to VA's comprehensive medical benefits package, certain benefits may vary from individual to individual, depending on each Veteran's unique eligibility status. The following care services (partial listing) have limitations and may have special eligibility criteria:

- Ambulance Services
- Dental Care
- Non-VA Health Care Services

## Hearing Aids and Eyeglasses

Hearing aids, contact lenses and eyeglasses may be provided to the following enrolled Veterans as authorized in 38 CFR , provided they are receiving VA care or services:

- Veterans with any compensable service connected disability

- Former Prisoner of War (POWs)

- Veterans awarded a Purple Heart

- Veterans in receipt of benefits under 38 USC 1151 (i.e. Benefits for persons disabled by treatment or vocational rehabilitation).

- Veterans in receipt of increased pension based on the need for aid and attendance benefits or by reason of being permanently housebound

- Veterans who have a visual or hearing impairment resulting from the existence of another medical condition for which the Veteran is receiving VA care or which resulted from treatment of that medical condition

- Veterans with significant functional or cognitive impairment evidenced by deficiencies in activities of daily living (not including normally occurring visual or hearing impairments)

- Veterans with severe visual or hearing impairment and hearing aids and/or eyeglasses are necessary to ensure the Veteran's active participation in their own medical treatment

- Veterans with a 0% service connected hearing disability

Marines with II Marine Expeditionary Force returned to Marine Corps Air Station New River, North Carolina, from a deployment to Afghanistan in support of Operation Enduring Freedom, Dec. 6, 2014. HMLA-467 was part of the last Marines to be deployed to the Helmand province of Afghanistan in support of OEF with the purpose of providing close-air support to the Marines operating on the ground. (U.S. Marine Corps photo by Lance Cpl. Olivia McDonald/ Released)

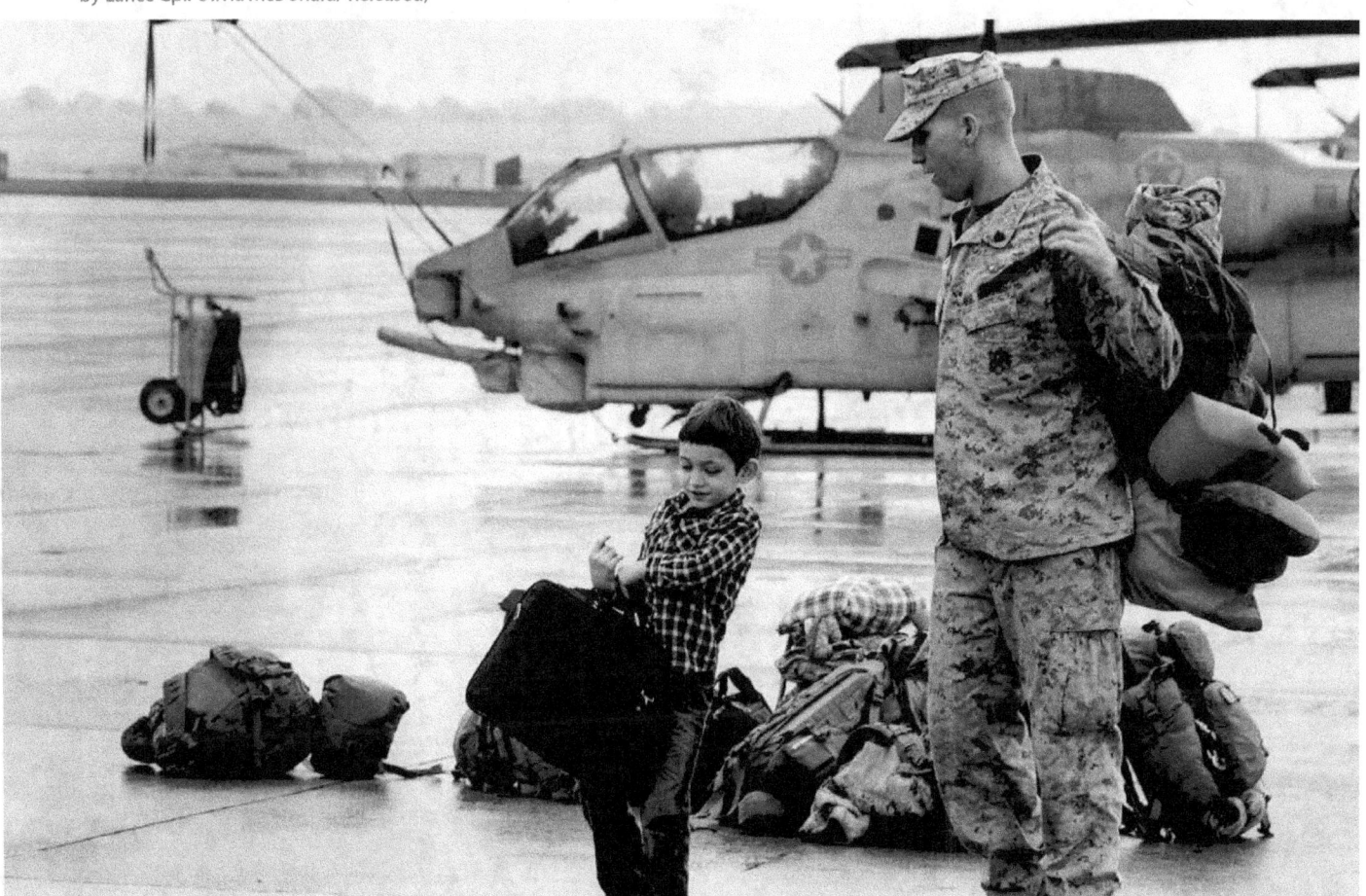

Your VA & DoD Benefits. Online.
Register Now
www.ebenefits.va.gov
"I just checked my Post-9/11 GI Bill enrollment. Online."
Your time is valuable. When you need fast, easy access to manage your VA & DoD benefits, claims and military documents, go online and register for a Premium eBenefits Account at www.ebenefits.va.gov.
eBenefits
www.ebenefits.va.gov

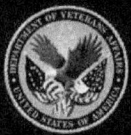

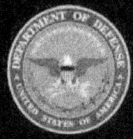

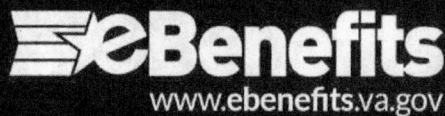

# Additional VA Health Benefits Programs
## Dependents and Survivors

### CHAMPVA

A health care benefits program for:

- Dependents of Veterans who have been rated by VA as having a service-connected total and permanent disability.
- Survivors of Veterans who died from VA-rated service-connected condition(s), or who at the time of death, were rated permanently and totally disabled from a VA-rated service-connected condition(s).
- Survivors of persons who died in the line of duty and not due to misconduct and not otherwise entitled to benefits under DoD's TRICARE program.

| Address | Telephone | Have Questions? |
|---|---|---|
| CHAMPVA<br>PO Box 469063<br>Denver, CO 80246-9063 | 800-733-8387 | https://iris.custhelp.com/ |

| CHAMPVA online |
|---|
| www.va.gov/purchasedcare/programs/dependents/champva/index.asp |

### Children of Women Vietnam Veterans Health Care Benefits

A program designed for women Vietnam Veterans' birth children who are determined by a VA Regional Office to have one or more covered birth defects.

| Address | Telephone | Have Questions? |
|---|---|---|
| Children of Women Vietnam Veterans<br>PO Box 469065<br>Denver, CO  80246-9065 | 888-820-1756 | https://iris.custhelp.com/ |

| CWVV online |
|---|
| www.va.gov/PURCHASEDCARE/programs/dependents/cwvv/index.asp |

### Spina Bifida Health Care Benefits

A program designed for certain birth children of Vietnam and Korea Veterans' birth children diagnosed with spina bifida and who are in receipt of a VA Regional Office award for spina bifida benefits.

| Address | Telephone | Have Questions? |
|---|---|---|
| Spina Bifida Health Care<br>PO Box 469065<br>Denver, CO  80246-9065 | 888-820-1756 | https://iris.custhelp.com/ |

| Spina Bifida online |
|---|
| www.va.gov/PURCHASEDCARE/programs/dependents/spinabifida/index.asp |

# Emergency Care

A medical emergency is generally defined as a condition of such a nature that a sensible person would reasonably expect that a delay in seeking immediate medical attention would be hazardous to life or health.

You may receive emergency care at a non-VA health care facility, possibly at VA expense, when a VA facility (or other Federal health care facility with which VA has an agreement) cannot furnish efficient care due to your distance from the facility; or when VA is unable to furnish the needed emergency services.

## VA Payment for Emergency Care of your Service-connected conditions without prior authorization

Since payment may be limited to the point when your condition is stable enough for you to travel to a VA facility, you or a family member or friend need to contact the nearest VA medical facility as soon as possible.  An emergency is deemed to have ended at the point when a VA provider has determined that, based on sound medical judgment, you could be transferred from the non-VA facility to a VA medical center.

VA may pay for your non-VA emergency care:

| If you are: | Then: |
| --- | --- |
| Service-connected | • VA may pay for your non-VA emergency care for a rated service-connected disability, or |
| | • Your nonservice-connected condition associated with and held to be aggravating your service-connected condition, or |
| | • Any condition, if you are an active participant in the VA Chapter 31 Vocational Rehabilitation program, and you need treatment to make possible your entrance into a course of training or to prevent interruption of a course of training, or |
| | • Any condition, if you are rated as having a total disability permanent in nature resulting from your service-connected disability, or |
| | • Other approved reason |

**VA Payment for Emergency Care of your NonService-connected conditions without prior authorization**

VA may pay for emergency care provided in a non-VA facility for treatment of a Non service-connected condition only if all of the following conditions are met:

| If you are: | Then: |
|---|---|
| Service-connected, not Permanently and Totally Disabled, or Nonservice-connected | VA may pay for your non-VA emergency care for treatment of a Nonservice-connected condition if all of the following conditions are met: <br><br>• The episode of care cannot be paid under another VA authority, and <br><br>• Based on an average knowledge of health and medicine (prudent layperson standard) you reasonably expected that delay in seeking immediate medical attention would have been hazardous to your life or health, and <br><br>• A VA or other Federal facility/provider was not feasibly available, and <br><br>• You received VA medical care within a 24-month period preceding the non-VA emergency care, and <br><br>• You are financially liable to the health care provider for the emergency care, and <br><br>• The services were furnished by an Emergency Department or similar facility held out to provide emergency care to the general public, and <br><br>• You have no other coverage under a health plan (including Medicare, Medicaid and Worker's Compensation), and <br><br>• You have no contractual or legal recourse against a third party that would, in whole, extinguish your liability |

# VA Dental Insurance Program (VADIP)

VA would like all Veterans to have access to good oral health care; however, VA is limited to providing dental benefits to those Veterans who meet certain eligibility criteria.

VA offers enrolled Veterans and beneficiaries of VA's Civilian Health and Medical Program (CHAMPVA), the opportunity to purchase dental insurance at a reduced cost. VA is making this special benefit available through Delta Dental and MetLife via a pilot program. Multiple options allow participants to select a plan that provides benefits and premiums that meet their dental needs and budget. Each enrollee will pay a fixed monthly premium for coverage, in addition to any copayments required by his or her plan.

There are no eligibility limitations based on service-connected disability rating or enrollment priority assignment. People interested in participating in this pilot program may complete an application online through either the websites of Delta Dental, www.deltadentalvadip.org, or MetLife, www.metlife.com/VADIP. Coverage for this new dental insurance is available throughout the United States and its territories.

For more information about this program, call 1-877-222-VETS (8387) between 8AM and 8PM ET, Monday – Friday, or visit www.va.gov/healthbenefits/vadip, and click the insurers' link for specific information regarding registration, premiums and services.

# Mental Health Services

## Military Sexual Trauma

Military Sexual Trauma (MST) is the term VA uses to refer to sexual assault or repeated, threatening sexual harassment occurring during a Veteran's military service. VA has expanded eligibility for Veterans in need of mental health care due to sexual assault or sexual harassment to Reservists and National Guard members participating in weekend drill. Veterans can learn more about VA's MST-related services online at www.mentalhealth.va.gov/msthome.asp.

## In-/outpatient and Residential Services Available

VA provides free outpatient, inpatient, and residential services to assist Veterans in their recovery from MST. MST services are available to both male and female Veterans without a limit to the duration of care. MST-related outpatient services are available at every VA health care facility. VA also has programs that offer specialized MST treatment in a residential or inpatient setting. These programs are for those who need more intense treatment and support.

## Receive Free MST-Related Care

To receive free treatment related to MST, Veterans do not need a VA service-connected disability. Veterans do not need to have reported the incident when it happened or have other documentation that it occurred. There are no length–of–service requirements to receive care, and some Veterans may be able to receive free MST-related care even if they are not eligible for other VA care.

For more information, please contact the MST Coordinator at your nearest VA Medical Center or visit www.mentalhealth.va.gov/msthome.asp. A list of VA and Vet Center facilities can be found online at www.va.gov/directory/.

## Readjustment Counseling Services

VA provides free readjustment counseling and outreach services to Veterans who served in a theater of operations (combat zone), through community based counseling centers called Vet Centers. Services are also available for their family members for military related issues. Vet Center staffs are available toll-free during normal business hours at 1-800-905-4675 (ET) and 1-866-496-8838 (PT). For information online, visit www.vetcenter.va.gov.

# Veterans Crisis Line

The Veterans Crisis Line is a toll-free, confidential resource that connects Veterans in crisis and their families and friends with qualified, caring VA responders.

Veterans and their loved ones can **call 1-800-273-8255 and Press 1, chat online at** www.veteranscrisisline. net, or send a **text message to 838255** to receive confidential support 24 hours a day, 7 days a week, 365 days a year, ***even if they are not registered with VA or enrolled in VA health care***.

The professionals at the Veterans Crisis Line are specially trained and experienced in helping Veterans of all ages and circumstances — from Veterans coping with mental health issues that were never addressed to recent Veterans struggling with relationships or the transition back to civilian life.

# Homeless Veterans

VA has founded a National Call Center for Homeless Veterans to ensure that homeless Veterans or Veterans at -risk for homelessness have free, 24/7 access to trained counselors. The hotline is intended to assist homeless Veterans and their families, VA Medical Facilities, federal, state and local partners, community agencies, service providers and others in the community. To be connected with a trained VA staff member, call **1-877-4AID VET (877-424-3838).**

- Call for yourself or someone else
- Free and confidential
- Trained VA counselors to assist
- Available 24 hours a day, 7 days a week

Learn about VA homeless programs and mental health services in your area that can help you. For more information, visit www.va.gov/homeless.

# Increasing Minority Veterans Participation

The goal of this program is to increase local awareness of minority Veteran related issues and encourage eligible Veterans to participate in existing VA benefit programs and services. Minority Veteran Program Coordinators (MVPC) at each Health Care facility:

- Promote the use of VA benefits, programs, and services by minority Veterans.
- Support and initiate activities that educate and sensitize internal staff to the unique needs of minority Veterans.
- Target outreach efforts to minority Veterans through community networks.
- Advocate on behalf of minority Veterans by identifying gaps in services and make recommendations to improve service delivery within their facilities.

For more information and to locate the program coordinator in your area visit www.va.gov/centerforminorityveterans/Minority_Veterans_Programs_Coordinators_MVPC.asp.

# Caregivers Program

The caregivers benefit program provides certain medical, travel, training, and financial benefits to caregivers of certain Veterans and Servicemembers who were seriously injured during their military service on or after September 11, 2001. Eligible primary Family Caregivers can receive a stipend, training, mental health services, travel and lodging reimbursement, and access to health insurance if they are not already under a health care plan. For more information, contact your local VA medical facility and speak with a Caregiver Support Coordinator, visit www.caregiver.va.gov or dial toll-free 1-855-260-3274.

# Camp Lejeune Water Contamination Benefits

### Benefits have been extended to 1953

From the 1950s through the 1980s, people living or working at the U.S. Marine Corps Base Camp Lejeune, North Carolina, may have been exposed to drinking water contaminated with industrial solvents, benzene, and other chemicals.

Veterans who served on active duty at Camp Lejeune for at least 30 days between August 1, 1953 and December 31, 1987 may be eligible for cost-free medical care through VA for the following health conditions:

- Bladder cancer
- Breast cancer
- Esophageal cancer
- Female infertility
- Hepatic steatosis
- Kidney cancer
- Leukemia
- Lung cancer

- Miscarriage
- Multiple myeloma
- Myelodysplastic syndromes
- Neurobehavioral effects
- Non-Hodgkin's lymphoma
- Rena toxicity
- Scleroderma

Veterans already enrolled in VA health care should contact their local VA health care facility to receive care under the new law. Those not already enrolled should call 1-877-222-VETS (8387) for assistance. Family members will receive care after Congress appropriates funds and VA publishes regulations.

For further information about Camp Lejeune historical water contamination and to sign up for updates, visit the Military Exposure section on the VHA Office of Public Health website at www.publichealth.va.gov/exposures.

The U.S. Marine Corps encourages all those who lived or worked at Camp Lejeune before 1987 to register to receive notifications regarding Camp Lejeune Historic Drinking Water at https://clnr.hqi.usmc.mil/clwater/.

# Medically Related Travel Benefits

Veterans may qualify for mileage reimbursement or special mode transportation in relation to travel for VA health care if they:

- Have a service-connected disability rating of 30 percent or more; or
- Are traveling for treatment of a service-connected condition; or
- Receive a VA pension; or
- Are traveling for a scheduled compensation or pension examination; or
- Have income below the maximum annual VA pension rate

Special mode travel (e.g., wheelchair van, ambulance) is provided to eligible Veterans based on a clinical determination of need (authorization is not required for emergencies if a delay would endanger their life or health).

Mileage Reimbursement of 41.5 cents per mile may be claimed to offset expense of travel when the Veteran drove to qualified appointment. Reimbursement for actual cost of common carrier travel (bus, train, taxi etc.) is available in some circumstances.

## No More Standing In Line

VA has implemented VA Form 10-3542 and created a simple way to apply for Mileage Reimbursement without standing in line. Contact your local VAMC Beneficiary Travel office for details.

Travel benefits are subject to a deductible. Exceptions to the deductible requirement include: 1) travel for a compensation and pension examination; 2) travel by an ambulance or a specially equipped van; and 3) when annual income does not exceed certain limits.

For more information on travel benefits, visit www.va.gov/HEALTHBENEFITS/vtp/Beneficiary_Travel.asp.

## Free Transportation To VA Appointments

VA recognizes Veterans who are visually impaired, elderly, or immobilized due to disease or disability, and particularly those living in remote and rural areas face challenges traveling to and from their VA health care facilities and authorized, non-VA health care appointments. To provide these Veterans with the most convenient and timely access to transportation services, VA is establishing a network of community transportation service providers that could include Veteran Service Organizations (VSOs); community and commercial transportation providers; federal, state and local government transportation services as well as non-profits, such as United We Ride.

Veterans needing transportation for care and treatment can contact their local VA medical center, patient travel office, for more information about the availability and types of service.

## Health Benefits For Service-Connected Conditions Are Never Out Of Reach

VA's Foreign Medical Program (FMP) provides health care benefits for U.S. Veterans with VA-rated service-connected conditions who are living or traveling abroad.

| All countries (excluding the Philippines) | | |
|---|---|---|
| **Address** | **Telephone** | **Fax** |
| Foreign Medical Program PO Box 469061 Denver, CO 80246-9061 | 303-331-7590 | 303-331-7803 |
| **To contact FMP online** | **Web site** | |
| https://iris.custhelp.com/ | www.va.gov/PURCHASEDCARE/programs/veterans/fmp | |

| Medical Services in the Philippines | | |
|---|---|---|
| **Address** | **Phone** | **Fax** |
| VA Outpatient Clinic – Manila Department of Veterans Affairs PSC 501 DPO, AP 96515 | 1-800-1888-8782 or 011-632-318-VETS (8387) | 011-632-310-5957 |

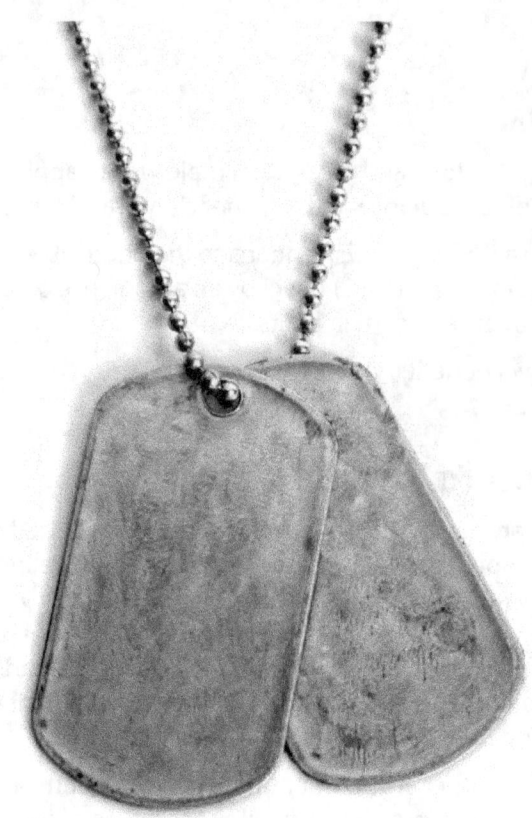

# Our Mission

Our Servicemembers and Veterans have sacrificed to keep our country - and everything it represents - safe.  We honor and serve those men and women by fulfilling President Lincoln's promise *"to care for him who shall have borne the battle, and for his widow, and his orphan."*

We strive to provide Servicemembers and Veterans with the world-class benefits and services they have earned, and will adhere to the highest standards of compassion, commitment, excellence, professionalism, integrity, accountability, and stewardship.

Thank you for your service.
Now let us serve you.

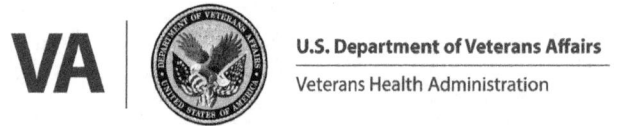

**U.S. Department of Veterans Affairs**
Veterans Health Administration

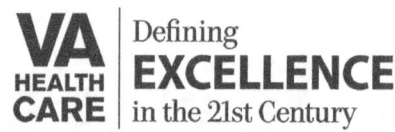

VA
HEALTH
CARE

Defining
**EXCELLENCE**
in the 21st Century

# Notice of Privacy Practices

Veterans who are enrolled for VA health care benefits have various privacy rights under federal law and regulations, including the right to a Notice of Privacy Practices. To review the VA Notice of Privacy Practices, visit www.oprm.va.gov/privacy/resources_privacy.aspx or write to the VHA Privacy Office (19F2), 810 Vermont Avenue NW, Washington, DC 20420.

# Services and Tools Available Online

## VA's Health Benefits website

VA's health benefits website, located at www.va.gov/healthbenefits, contains a wide range of information related to the medical benefits, information and resources available to its enrollees, such as:

- Online application for enrollment
- Newly-released information regarding updates or changes to VA health care benefits and services
- Medical benefits based on eligibility and priority group
- Eligibility and benefits determination calculator
- Copay information
- Contact Information
- Online chat features
- Access to downloadable resources (fact sheets, brochures, etc.)
- Resource library
- Links to other sites of interest, such as MyHealtheVet, eBenefits, Pay.gov and the Affordable Care Act.

## Office of Public Health

The VA Office of Public Health brings a public health approach to promoting and protecting the health of Veterans and VA staff. Visit www.publichealth.va.gov to learn about important health related subjects including:

### Health & Wellness

- Topics that cover staying healthy with vaccinations and infection- control habits, employee wellness programs, and violence prevention

### Diseases & Conditions

- Find out more about certain medical conditions that may affect Veterans

### VA conducted health related studies and data

- The Office of Public Health and research organizations conduct studies on the health issues affecting Veterans to better serve their needs

### Military Exposures

- Learn about Exposure related health concerns

## Self-Service Kiosks

VA offers touch-screen devices at VA Medical Centers (VAMCs) and Community Based Outpatient Centers (CBOCs) for Veterans to have convenient control and access to health information.  Activities include:

- Check in for and view future appointments
- Manage, review and update personal and insurance information
- Apply for beneficiary travel mileage reimbursement
- Request medical records
- Manage account balance
- Review and reconcile medication and allergy information

More capabilities will be available soon.  Visit www.va.gov/healthbenefits/vps to learn more.

Sgt. Irene Lopez, 13th Expeditionary Sustainment Command, shares a touching moment with her daughter following the welcome home ceremony, Dec. 9, for 126 soldiers of the 13th ESC as they returned home from a yearlong deployment in Afghanistan.

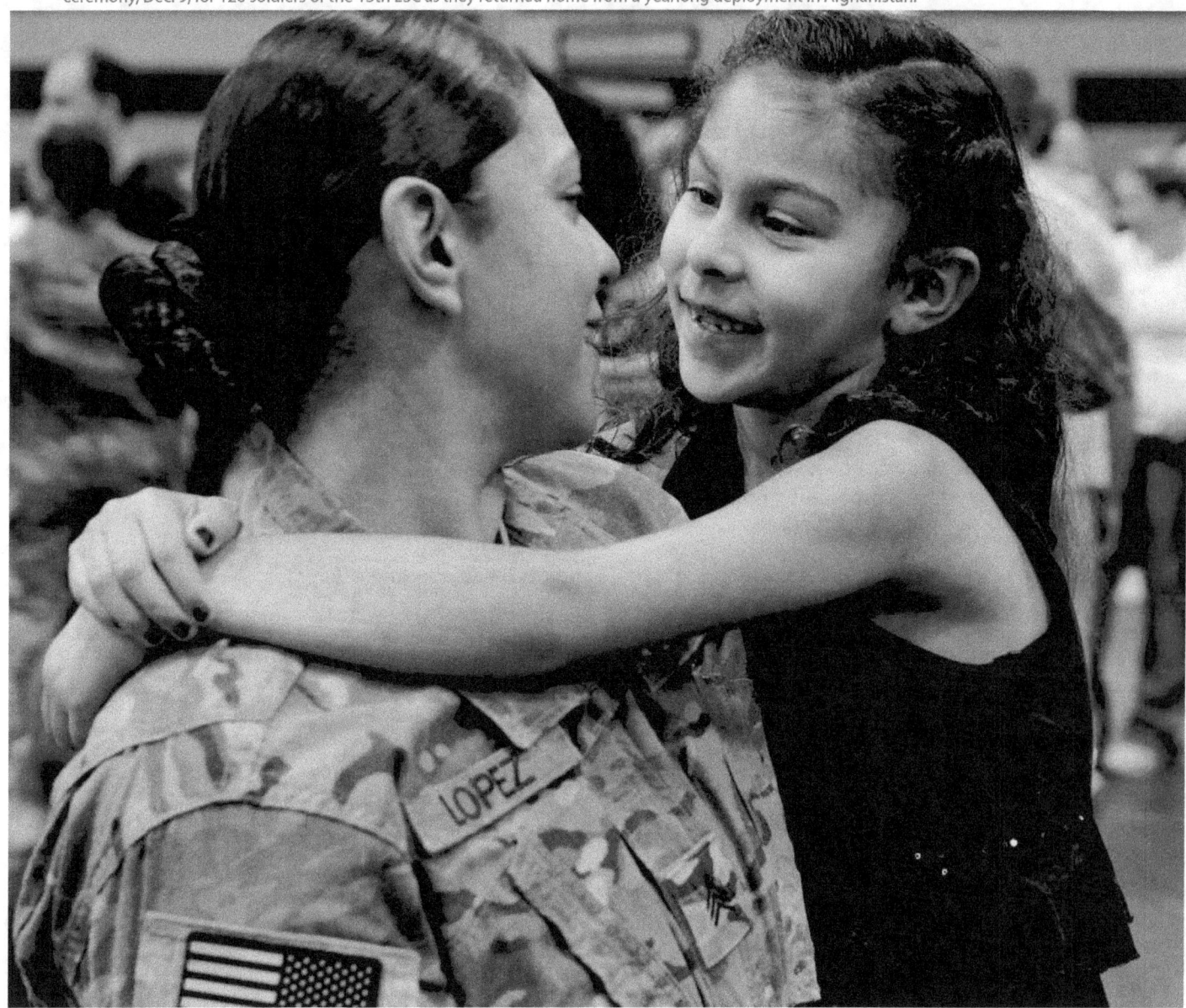

# Your Personal VA Health Information At Your Finger Tips

## MyHealtheVet

VA emphasizes patient-centered innovations including MyHealtheVet (www.myhealth.va.gov), an e-portal suite of tools for Veterans and Caregivers that provides a secure web-based Personal Health Record (PHR), patient access to personal health information from the VA Electronic Health Record, the ability to download and share personal health information using the VA Blue Button, online services such as e-prescription refills, trusted health education resources, and Secure Messaging between patients and their VA health care teams.

If you are a VA patient and have an upgraded account (obtained by completing the one-time Authentication process), you can:

- Participate in Secure Messaging with your participating VA health care team members
- Request prescription refills
- View key portions of your Department of Defense (DOD) Military Service Information
- Get your VA Wellness Reminders
- View your VA Appointments
- View your VA Lab Results
- View your VA Allergies and Adverse Reactions and other key portions of their VA electronic record
- View your VA Comprehensive Care Document (CCD)
    - o PLUS, participate in future features as they become available

Visit MyHealtheVet at www.myhealth.va.gov, register and learn more about authentication PLUS the many features and tools available to you 24/7 anywhere you have Internet access.  If you have any questions about MyHealtheVet, contact the MyHealtheVet Coordinator at your local VA facility.

## Special Care Access Network –
## Extension for Community Healthcare Outcomes (SCAN-ECHO)

Through VA's SCAN-ECHO initiative, Veterans and their primary care team use videoconferencing technology to seek expertise from specialists located 100-500 miles away.  VA offers SCAN ECHO to more than 40 rural sites of care with more than 100 participating rural primary care physicians, nurse practitioners, and physician assistants.

## Mobile Apps

VA is leveraging mobile health technology to provide Veterans with additional opportunities to become active partners in their health care.  VA Mobile releases new Apps for Veterans regularly. Check https://mobile.va.gov/ often for new information about available Apps.

## eBenefits

eBenefits is a one-stop shop for benefits-related information for Veterans, Wounded Warriors, Service Members, their families, and their caretakers. eBenefits allows Veterans to apply for VA benefits, such as health care, education and pension. Other services include:

**APPLY –**

- Disability Compensation
- Add or Remove Dependent
- VA Health Care
- Education Benefits

**MANAGE BENEFITS –**

- Compensation Claims Status
- Upload Supporting Documents for compensation claims
- Direct Deposit
- VA Letters

**MANAGE HEALTH –**

- VA Medical Records
- VA Prescription Refills
- VA Appointment Scheduling
- Order Hearing Aid Batteries

For additional information, please visit: www.ebenefits.va.gov.

## Veterans Canteen Service

Veterans Canteen Service (VCS) offers you the opportunity to shop and dine at any of its store/café operations located in VA hospitals and in many Community Outpatient Clinics across the country and in some Veterans Benefits Offices. The VCS Patriot Store Direct 1-800 Special Order program offers savings on top name brand retail items, such as computers, tires, tools, large appliances, flowers, jewelry, toys and much more. Browse vendors and monthly features at www.vacanteen.va.gov/PatriotStoreHome.php or call 1-800-664-8258 to place an order Monday – Friday 8AM – 6PM ET. For more information, visit www.vacanteen.va.gov.

# Frequently Asked Questions

### What is the Clay Hunt Act?
The Clay Hunt Suicide Prevention for American Veterans Act, which was signed into law February 12, 2015, provides a one-year window of enhanced VA health care enrollment for non-enrolled combat Veterans who were discharged or released from active military, naval, or air service after January 1, 2009, and before January 1, 2011.

### Where can I find more information?
Call our toll-free help line at 1-877-222-VETS (8387), Monday through Friday between 8AM and 8PM, ET. Information is also available at www.va.gov/healthbenefits.

### How can I verify my enrollment?
Once your enrollment is confirmed, you will receive a Veterans Health Benefits Handbook from us notifying you of the status of your enrollment. You may also call us to verify your enrollment at 1-877-222-VETS (8387) between 8AM and 8PM ET, Monday – Friday.

### If enrolled, must I use VA as my exclusive health care provider?
There is no requirement that VA become your exclusive provider of care. If you are a Veteran who is receiving care from both a VA provider and a local provider, it is important for your health and safety that your care from both providers is coordinated, resulting in one treatment plan (co-managed care).

### I am moving to another state. How do I transfer my care to a new VA health care facility?
If you want to transfer your care from one VA health care facility to another, contact the Enrollment Office for assistance in transferring your care and establishing an appointment at the new facility.

### How do I choose a preferred facility? How do I change my preferred facility?
When you apply for enrollment, you will be asked to choose a preferred VA facility. This will be the VA facility where you will receive your primary care. You may select any VA facility that is convenient for you. If the facility you choose cannot provide the health care that you need, VA will make other arrangements for your care, based on administrative eligibility and medical necessity. If you do not choose a preferred facility, VA will choose the facility that is closest to your home. You may change your preferred facility at anytime.

### Can I cancel my VA health care coverage?
Yes. You can submit a signed document stating that you no longer wish to be enrolled. Mail it to:

> Health Eligibility Center
> Enrollment Eligibility Division
> 2957 Clairmont Road Suite 200
> Atlanta, GA 30329-1647

However, acceptance for future VA health care coverage will be based on laws in place and your eligibility at the time of application should you reapply.

### Where can I find the new income limits?
Because the VA income limits may change each year, they are not published in this booklet. However, the income limit tables can be viewed on-line at www.va.gov/healthbenefits/cost.

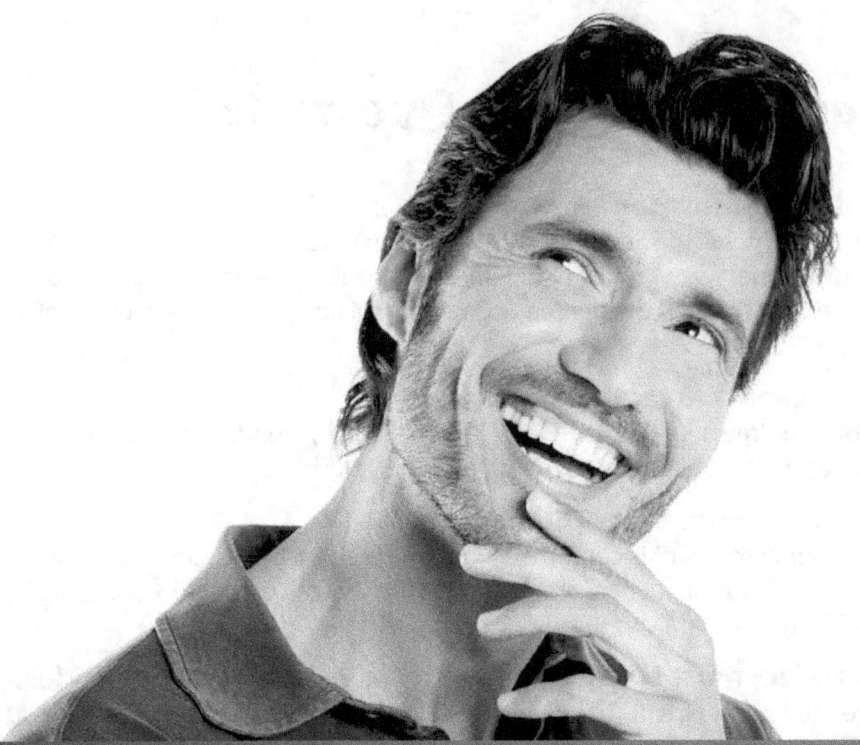

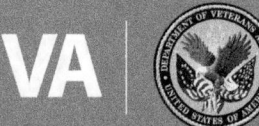

## What is a geographic income limit?

Recognizing the cost of living can vary significantly from one geographic area to another, Congress added income limits based on geographic locations to the existing VA income limits for financial assessment purposes. Those Veterans whose income falls between the VA income limit limits and the geographic income limit for the Veteran's locale will have their inpatient medical care copayments reduced by 80%. Geographic income limits can be found at www.va.gov/healthbenefits/cost/income_thresholds.asp.

## What happens if at the end of the process my income is verified to be higher than the income limits?

Your copay status will be changed from copay exempt to copay required, which may result in a disenrollment due to enrollment restrictions for Veterans whose income exceeds the income limits. VA facilities involved in your care will be notified of your change in status and to initiate billing for services provided during that income year. Your enrollment priority status may be changed if your financial status is adjusted by the income verification (IV) process. If your enrollment status is changed, you will be notified by mail.

## Does VA have access to my income tax return?

No, VA does not have access to your tax return. The Internal Revenue Service (IRS) and the Social Security Administration (SSA) share earned and unearned income data reported by employers and financial institutions.

## I am a recently discharged combat Veteran. Must I pay VA copayments?

Veterans who qualify under this special eligibility are not subject to copayments for conditions potentially related to their combat service. However, unless otherwise exempted, combat Veterans must either disclose their prior year gross household income OR decline to provide their financial information and agree to make applicable copayments for care or services VA determines are clearly unrelated to their military service.

If the services are provided for the treatment of a condition that may be potentially related to your military service in a theater of combat operations, you will not be charged any copayments.

## What is a VA service-connected rating, and how do I establish one?

A service-connected rating is an official ruling by VA that your illness or condition is directly related to your active military service. To obtain more information or to apply for any of these benefits, contact your nearest VA Regional Office at 1-800-827-1000, visit www.ebenefits.va.gov, or visit us online at www.va.gov.

## What if I receive a bill and cannot pay?

If you are unable to pay your bill, you should discuss the matter with the Patient Billing Office at the VA health care facility where you received your care. There are four possible options that may be available to you:

**Hardship Determination** – If a Veteran's current year income is substantially reduced from the prior year. Future exemption from medical and hospital care copayments for a determined period of time. (See your facilities Enrollment Coordinator for Hardship consideration.)

**Waiver** – If there has been a significant change in income or significant expenses for medical care for the Veteran or other family members, funeral arrangements or Veteran educational expenses. A waiver is for past debts only. (See your local Patient Billing Office staff for additional information.)

**Offer in Compromise** – Offer for past debts only and acceptance of a partial payment in settlement and full satisfaction of debt. (See your local Patient Billing Office staff for additional information.)

**Repayment Plans** – Payment of past debt generally over a period of 36 months. (See your local revenue staff for additional information.)

You must contact the facility at which you received the care to request one of these options.

## What is the Affordable Care Act?

The Affordable Care Act, also known as the health care law, was created to expand access to affordable health care coverage to all Americans, lower costs, and improve quality and care coordination. For more information, visit www.va.gov/aca.

## If I am enrolled in VA Health care, do I meet the requirements for health care coverage?

Yes. If you are enrolled in any of VA's programs below, you have coverage under the standards of the health care law:

- Veteran's health care program
- Civilian Health and Medical program (CHAMPVA)
- Spina bifida health care program

## When do I begin declaring health care coverage to Internal Revenue Service (IRS)?

Starting in 2015, U.S. taxpayers will need to declare that they have health coverage on their federal tax forms. IRS does not require any specific forms to report health coverage in 2015.

## Do I need to report to IRS that I had health care coverage in 2014?

Yes. Line 61 on Internal Revenue Service Form 1040, Line 38 on the 1040A and various other entries on IRS income tax forms require taxpayers to self-declare whether they had health care coverage in 2014.

## When will VA begin notifying the Internal Revenue Service (IRS) of a Veteran's enrollment in the VA health care system?

Starting in 2016, VA will send IRS, Veterans and eligible beneficiaries forms that provide details of the health coverage provided by VA. These forms are to be used for the income tax process. This year, in 2015, no forms are needed to complete the income tax process.

## What is a PACT?

A Patient Aligned Care Team (PACT) is each Veteran working together with health care professionals to plan for the whole-person care and life-long health and wellness. They focus on:

- Partnerships with Veterans
- Access to care using diverse methods
- Coordinated care among team members
- Team-based care with Veterans as the center of their PACT

## How does a PACT function?

A PACT uses a team-based approach. You are the center of the care team that also includes your family members, caregivers and your health care professionals—primary care provider, nurse care manager, clinical associate, and administrative clerk. When other services are needed to meet your goals and needs, another care team may be called in. For more information visit www.va.gov/health/services/primarycare/pact/.

## Am I eligible for dental care?

Dental benefits are provided by the VA according to law. In some instances, VA is authorized to provide extensive dental care, while in other cases treatment may be limited. The Chart below describes dental eligibility criteria and contains information to assist Veterans in understanding their eligibility for VA dental care.

The eligibility for outpatient dental care is not the same as for most other VA medical benefits and is categorized into classes. For instance, if you are eligible for VA dental care under Class I, IIC, or IV you are eligible for any necessary dental care to maintain or restore oral health and masticatory function, including repeat care. Other classes have time and/or service limitations.

The Chart below describes dental eligibility criteria and contains information to assist Veterans in understanding their eligibility for VA dental care.

| If you: | You are eligible for: |
|---------|----------------------|
| Have a service-connected compensable dental disability or condition. | Any needed dental care. |
| Are a former prisoner of war. | Any needed dental care. |
| Have service-connected disabilities rated 100% disabling, or are unemployable and paid at the 100% rate due to service-connected conditions. | Any needed dental care.<br><br>[**Please note:** Veterans paid at the 100% rate based on a temporary rating, such as extended hospitalization for a service-connected disability, convalescence or pre-stabilization are not eligible for comprehensive outpatient dental services based on this temporary rating]. |
| Apply for dental care within 180 days of discharge or release from a period of active duty (under conditions other than dishonorable) of 90 days or more during the Persian Gulf War era. | One-time dental care if your DD 214 certificate of discharge does not indicate that a complete dental examination and all appropriate dental treatment had been rendered prior to discharge.* |
| Have a service-connected noncompensable dental condition or disability resulting from combat wounds or service trauma. | Any dental care necessary to provide and maintain a functioning dentition. A Dental Trauma Rating (VA Form 10-564-D) or VA Regional Office Rating Decision letter (VA Form 10-7131) identifies the tooth/teeth that are trauma rated. |
| Have a dental condition clinically determined by VA to be associated with and aggravating a service-connected medical condition. | Dental care to treat the oral conditions that are determined by a VA dental professional to have a direct and material detrimental effect to your service connected medical condition. |

| If you: | You are eligible for: |
|---|---|
| Are actively engaged in a 38 USC Chapter 31 vocational rehabilitation program | Dental care to the extent necessary as determined by a VA dental professional to:<br><br>• Make possible your entrance into a rehabilitation program<br><br>• Achieve the goals of your vocational rehabilitation program<br><br>• Prevent interruption of your rehabilitation program<br><br>• Hasten the return to a rehabilitation program if you are in interrupted or leave status<br><br>• Hasten the return to a rehabilitation program of a Veteran placed in discontinued status because of illness, injury or a dental condition, or<br><br>• Secure and adjust to employment during the period of employment assistance, or enable you to achieve maximum independence in daily living. |
| Are receiving VA care or are scheduled for inpatient care and require dental care for a condition complicating a medical condition currently under treatment. | Dental care to treat the oral conditions that are determined by a VA dental professional to complicate your medical condition currently under treatment. |
| Are an enrolled Veteran who may be homeless and receiving care under VHA Directive 2007-039. | A one-time course of dental care that is determined medically necessary to relieve pain, assist you to gain employment, or treat moderate, severe, or complicated and severe gingival and periodontal conditions. |

**\* Note:** Public Law 83 enacted June 16, 1955, amended Veterans' eligibility for outpatient dental services. As a result, any Veteran who received a dental award letter from VBA dated before 1955 in which VBA determined the dental conditions to be noncompensable are no longer eligible for Class II outpatient dental treatment.

Veterans receiving hospital, nursing home, or domiciliary care will be provided dental services that are professionally determined by a VA dentist, in consultation with the referring physician, to be essential to the management of the patient's medical condition under active treatment.

For more information about eligibility for VA medical and dental benefits, contact VA at 1-877-222-VETS (8387) or www.va.gov/healthbenefits.

## What is Non-VA Care?

Non-VA care is when the Veteran's VA care team determines that the Veteran should be referred to a Non-VA provider and the VA would pay for the cost of that care because:

- Demand exceeds VA health care facility capacity
- Need for diagnostic support services for VA clinicians
- Need for scarce specialty resources (e.g., obstetrics, hyperbaric, burn care, oncology) and/or when VA resources are not available due to constraints (e.g. staffing, space)
- Ensure cost-effectiveness for VA
- Outside procurement vs. maintaining and operating like services in VA facilities for infrequent use
- To satisfy patient wait-time requirements

## Do I qualify for routine health care at non-VA facilities at VA expense?

Generally no. To qualify for routine care at non-VA facilities at VA expense you must first be given a written referral. Included among the factors in determining whether such care will be authorized is your medical condition and availability of VA services within your geographic area. VA copayments may be applicable.

## Am I eligible for emergency care at a non-VA facility?

An eligible Veteran may receive emergency care at a non-VA health care facility at VA expense when a VA facility or other Federal health care facility with which VA has an agreement is unable to furnish economical care due to the Veteran's geographical inaccessibility to a VA medical facility, or when VA is unable to furnish the needed emergency services. (See Emergency Care on page 28 for specific rules)

## Are there any payment limitations for non-VA emergency care?

Emergency care must be pre-authorized by VA. When the emergency care is not authorized in advance by VA, it may be considered as preauthorized care when the nearest VA medical facility is notified within 72 hours of admission, the Veteran is eligible, and the care rendered is emergent in nature. Claims for non-VA emergency care not authorized by VA in advance of services being furnished must be timely filed; because timely filing requirements differ by type of claim, you should contact the nearest VA medical facility as soon as possible to avoid payment denial for an untimely filed claim. (See Emergency Care on page 28 for specific rules)

Payment may not be approved for any period beyond the date on which the medical emergency ended, except when VA cannot accommodate transfer of the Veteran to a VA or other Federal facility. An emergency is deemed to have ended at that point when a VA physician has determined that, based on sound medical judgment, a Veteran who received emergency hospital care could have been transferred from the non-VA facility to a VA medical center for continuation of treatment.

## What type of emergency care can VA authorize in advance?

| Subject to eligibility and payment limitations described on page 28 (Emergency Care) , VA may preauthorize and issue payment for non-VA emergency care when treatment is needed for: | Inpatient Care | Outpatient Care |
|---|---|---|
| The Veteran's VA rated service-connected disability, or for a nonservice-condition that is associated with and aggravating the Veteran's service-connected condition | √ | √ |
| A disability for which the Veteran was released from active duty | √ | √ |
| Any condition of a Veteran who is rated by VA as Permanently and Totally disabled due to a service connected disability | √ | √ |
| Any condition of a Veteran who is an active participant in the VA Chapter 31 Vocational Rehabilitation program, who needs treatment medically determined to make possible the Veteran's entrance into a course of training, or prevent interruption of a course of training which was interrupted due to such illness, injury, or dental condition. | √ | √ |
| Any condition for a Veteran who has a VA service-connected disability rating of 50% or greater | | √ |
| A condition for which the Veteran has been furnished VA hospital care, nursing home, domiciliary care, or medical services and who requires medical services to complete treatment incident to such care or services | | √ |

| Subject to eligibility and payment limitations described on page 28 (Emergency Care) , VA may preauthorize and issue payment for non-VA emergency care when treatment is needed for: | Inpatient Care | Outpatient Care |
|---|---|---|
| Any condition of a Veteran who is in receipt of increased VA pension, or additional VA compensation or allowances based on the need for regular aid and attendance or by reason of being permanently housebound | | √ |
| A condition requiring emergency care that developed while the Veteran was receiving medical services in a VA facility or Contract Nursing Home or during VA authorized travel | √ | √ |
| Any condition that will obviate the need for hospital admission for a Veteran in the state of Alaska or Hawaii and US Territories, excluding Puerto Rico | | √ |
| Any condition for women Veterans. | √ | |
| Any dental services and treatment, and related dental appliances, for Veterans who are former prisoners of war | | √ |

## Can VA pay for non-VA emergency care that is not preauthorized?

VA has limited payment authority when emergency care at a non-VA facility is provided without authorization by VA in advance of services being furnished or notification to VA is not made within 72 hours of admission. VA may pay for unauthorized emergency care as indicated below. Since payment may be limited to the point your condition is stable for transfer to a VA facility, the nearest VA medical facility should be contacted as soon as possible for all care not authorized by VA in advance of the services being furnished.

| For service-connected Veterans | For Nonservice-connected conditions |
|---|---|
| VA may only pay for emergency care provided in a non-VA facility for certain Veterans who are rated by VA with a service-connected disability. VA may pay for emergency inpatient or outpatient care when treatment is needed for: | VA may only pay for emergency care provided in a non-VA facility for treatment of a Nonservice-connected condition only if **all** of the following conditions are met: |
| The Veteran's VA rated service connected disability, or for a nonservice-condition that is associated with and aggravating the Veteran's service-connected condition | The episode of care cannot be paid as an unauthorized claim for service-connected Veterans |
| A VA facility was not considered feasibly available when the urgency of the Veteran's medical condition, the relative distance of the travel involved, or the nature of the treatment required makes it necessary or economically advisable to use public or private facilities. | The Veteran is enrolled in the VHA health care system and received VA medical care within a 24 month period preceding the furnishing of the emergency treatment |
| Any condition of a Veteran who is rated by VA as Permanently and Totally disabled due to a service connected disability | The Veteran is personally liable to the health care provider for the emergency treatment which meets the prudent layperson definition of an emergency |

| For service-connected Veterans | For Nonservice-connected conditions |
|---|---|
| VA may only pay for emergency care provided in a non-VA facility for certain Veterans who are rated by VA with a service-connected disability. VA may pay for emergency inpatient or outpatient care when treatment is needed for: | VA may only pay for emergency care provided in a non-VA facility for treatment of a Nonservice-connected condition only if **all** of the following conditions are met: |
| Any condition of a Veteran who is an active participant in the VA Chapter 31 Vocational Rehabilitation program, who needs treatment medically determined to make possible the Veteran's entrance into a course of training, or prevent interruption of a course of training which was interrupted due to such illness, injury, or dental condition | The Veteran has no other contractual or legal recourse against a third party that would, in whole, extinguish the Veteran's liability and the claim must be filed within 90 days from the date of discharge, or the date that the Veteran exhausted without success action to obtain payment from a third party. |
| A prudent layperson would have reasonably expected that delay in seeking immediate medical attention would have been hazardous to life or health. | A prudent layperson would have reasonably expected that delay in seeking immediate medical attention would have been hazardous to life or health. |
| Once authorization for care is granted by VA, ,the authorization will be continued after admission only for the period of time required to stabilize or improve the patient's condition to the extent that further care is no longer required to satisfy the purpose for which it was initiated. | Once authorization for care is granted by VA, ,the authorization will be continued after admission only for the period of time required to stabilize or improve the patient's condition to the extent that further care is no longer required to satisfy the purpose for which it was initiated. |
|  | The Veteran is not entitled to care or services under a health plan contract |
|  | Treatment was provided in a hospital emergency room |

### Does VA offer compensation for travel expenses to and from a VA facility?

Yes, but not all Veterans qualify. If you meet specific criteria (see Medically Related Travel Benefits on page 32), you are eligible for travel benefits.

### I already provided financial information on my initial VA application, why is it necessary to complete a separate financial assessment for long-term care?

Unlike the information collected from the financial assessment, which is based on your previous year's income, the 10-10EC is designed to assess your current financial status, including current expenses. This in-depth analysis provides the necessary monthly income/expense information to determine whether you qualify for cost-free long-term care or a significant reduction from the maximum copay charge.

### Once I submit a completed VA Form 10-10EC, who notifies me of my long-term care copay requirements?

The social worker or case manager involved in your long-term care placement will provide you with an annual projection of your monthly copay charges.

## Assuming I qualify for nursing home care, how is it determined whether the care will be provided in a VA facility or a private nursing home at VA expense?

Generally, if you qualify for indefinite nursing home care, that care will be furnished in a VA facility. Care may be provided in a private facility under VA contract when there is compelling medical or social need.

If you do not qualify for indefinite care, you may be placed in a community nursing home—generally not to exceed six months—following an episode of VA care. The purpose of this short-term placement is to provide assistance to you and your families while alternative, long-term arrangements are explored.

## For Veterans who do not qualify for indefinite VA Community Living Center care at VA expense, what assistance is available for making alternative arrangements?

When the need for nursing home care extends beyond the Veteran's eligibility, our social workers will help family members identify possible sources for financial assistance. Our staff will review basic Medicare and Medicaid eligibility and direct the family to the appropriate sources for further assistance, including possible application for additional VA benefit programs.

### What does the new VHIC provide that the old ID card did not?

- Increased security for your personal information - no personally identifiable information is contained on the magnetic stripe or barcode.

- A salute to your military service – The emblem of your latest branch of service is displayed on your card. Several special awards will also be listed.

### What document(s) do I need to prove my identity to receive a Veteran Health Identification Card?

| Primary Identification | Secondary Identification |
|---|---|
| Present ONE form of Primary Identification | And ONE form of Secondary Identification |
| State-Issued Driver's License or ID | Social Security Card |
| U.S. Passport or U.S. Passport Card (unexpired) | Original or Certified Birth Certificate |
| Foreign passport with Form I-94 or Form I-94A (unexpired) | Certification of Birth Abroad Issued by the Department of State (Form FS-545) |
| U.S. Military card | Certification of Report of Birth issued by the Department of State (Form DS-1350) |
| Military dependent's ID card | Voter's Registration Card |
| U.S. Coast Guard Merchant Mariner Card | Native American Tribal Document |
| Foreign passport that contains a temporary I-551 stamp | U.S. Citizen ID Card (Form I-197) |
| Permanent Resident Card or Alien Registration Receipt Card (Form I- 551) | Identification Card for Use of Resident Citizen in the United States (Form I-179) |
| Federal, state, or local government issued ID card with a photograph | Employment Authorization document issued by the Department of Homeland Security |
| Employment Authorization Document that contains a photograph (Form I- 766) | Canadian Driver's License |

### What do I do if my VHIC is lost or stolen?

If your VHIC is lost or stolen, you should contact your local VA medical facility to get a new photo taken for a new card, or call us at 1-877- 222-VETS (8387).

# Notes

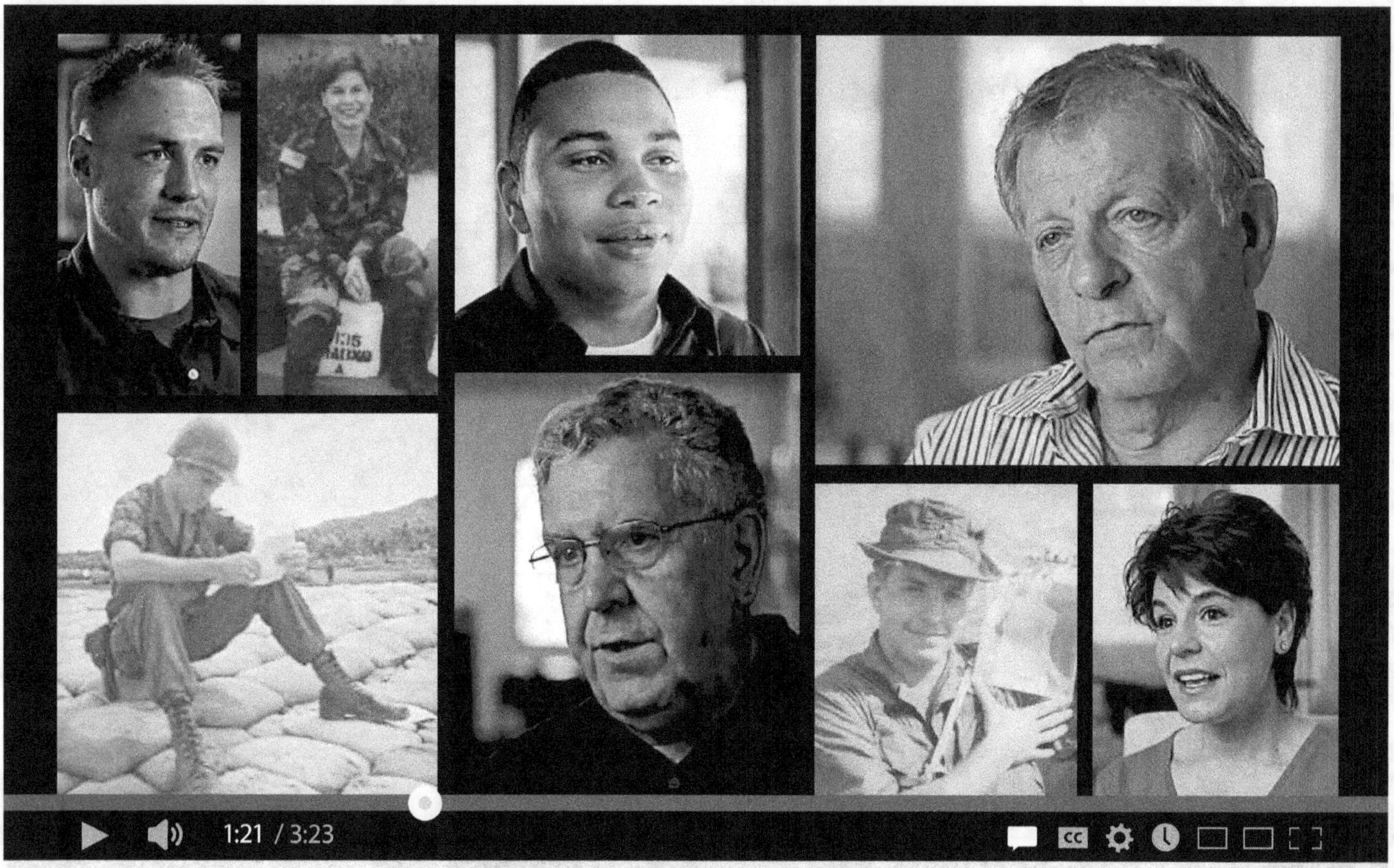

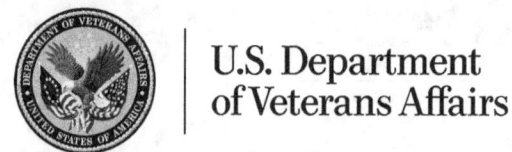
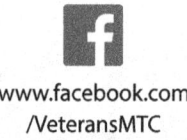
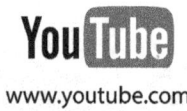
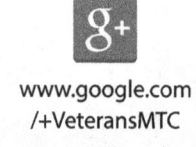

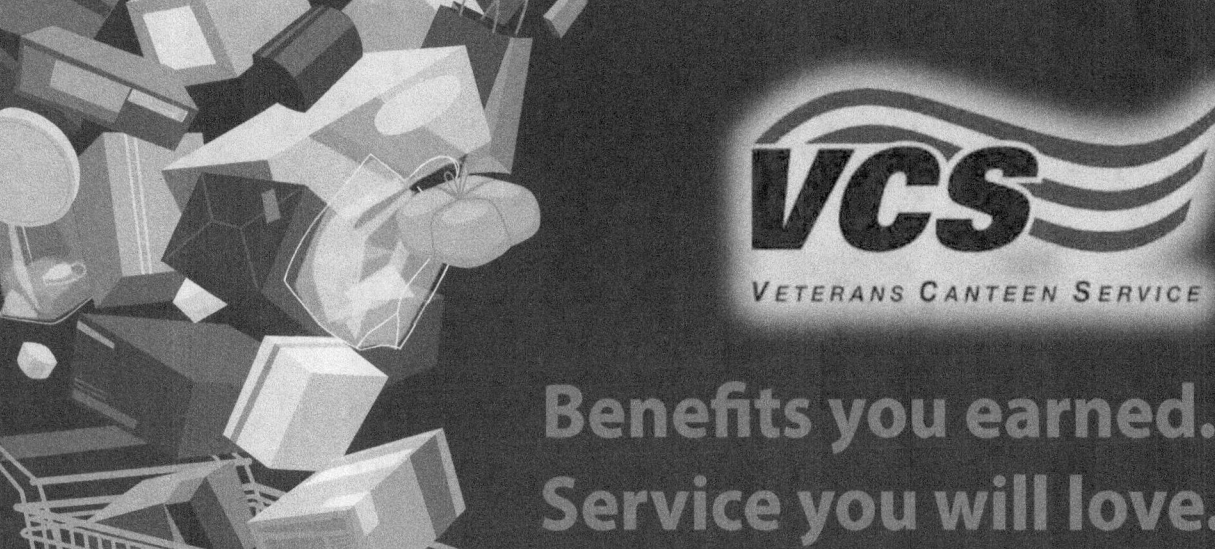

# Benefits you earned.
# Service you will love.

Our mission is to provide America's Veterans enrolled in VA's Healthcare System, their families, caregivers, VA employees, volunteers, and visitors, reasonably priced merchandise and services essential to their comfort and well-being.

Visit one of the 200+ convenient locations at your VA Medical Center. Shop your PatriotStore retail shop, enjoy breakfast or lunch in your PatriotCafé or grab a cup of coffee in your PatriotBrew.

Looking for something special? Check out your special order program, PatriotStoreDirect offering merchandise not sold in stores such as tires, flowers, computers, large appliances, jewelry, tools and toys. Call 1-800-664-8258 M-F 8:00 am – 6:00 pm EST to shop VCS special order.

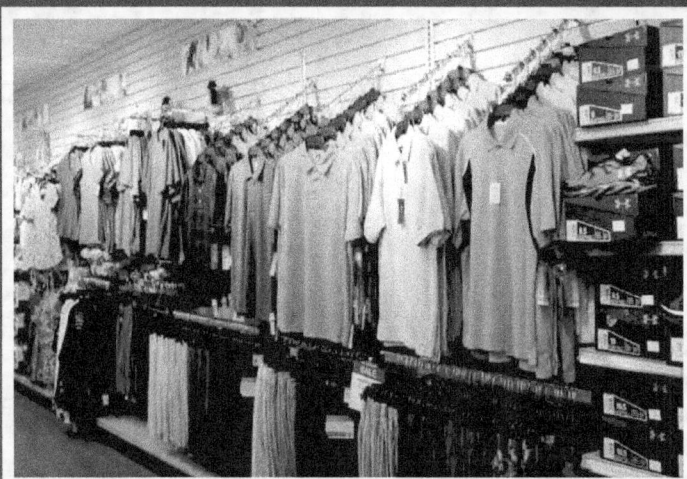

 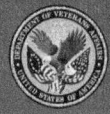 **U.S. Department of Veterans Affairs**
Veterans Health Administration

VCS is part of the Department of Veterans Affairs. It is a self-sustaining entity providing services only to authorized customers. Revenues generated from VCS are used to support a variety of programs such as: VA's Rehabilitation Games, Fisher Houses, Poly-Trauma Centers for OIF/OEF/OND Veterans, disaster relief efforts, VA's Homelessness initiatives, and other activities.

**Department of Veterans Affairs**
Veterans Health Administration
Chief Business Office

For more information on VA health care
Telephone (toll-free): 1-877-222-VETS (8387)
Website: www.va.gov/healthbenefits
To download a copy of this brochure, go to:
www.va.gov/healthbenefits/resources/epublications.asp

IB 10-185
Revised February 2015

www.ingramcontent.com/pod-product-compliance
Lightning Source LLC
Chambersburg PA
CBHW081421280526
45788CB00009B/3187